Remembering Yesterday, Caring Today

Reminiscence in Dementia Care
A Guide to Good Practice

Pam Schweitzer and Errollyn Bruce

Foreword by Faith Gibson

Jessica Kingsley *Publishers*
London and Philadelphia

First published in 2008
by Jessica Kingsley Publishers
116 Pentonville Road
London N1 9JB, UK
and
400 Market Street, Suite 400
Philadelphia, PA 19106, USA

www.jkp.com

Library of Congress Cataloging in Publication Data
A CIP catalog record for this book is available from the Library of Congress

British Library Cataloguing in Publication Data
A CIP catalogue record for this book is available from the British Library

ISBN 978 1 84310 649 4
eISBN 978 1 84642 804 3

Contents

Final Comments and Future Hopes   **193**

Photographs by Alex Schweitzer, Rado Klose
and Errollyn Bruce. (Unless otherwise stated,
the photographs in this book feature the London
RYCT groups.)

Foreword

This book is based on ten years of experience and experimenting with imaginative ways of involving people with dementia and those who share their lives as family members, friends, volunteers, and health and social care professionals in the riches of reminiscence work. The approach described and discussed here in vivid detail draws its strength from many sources and much practical experience. The use of ideas about person-centred care, so effectively developed and promulgated by Tom Kitwood, are woven together with the widening recognition of the centrality and value of using residual long-term memory, accessed by reminiscence and linked with various creative arts, to enrich the lives of everyone affected by dementia.

The Remembering Yesterday, Caring Today approach and projects which this book expounds had its antecedents in earlier conferences held at Age Exchange Reminiscence Centre, Blackheath, London. Visionary European Commission *fonctionnaires* Rosemarie Golz and Lars Rasmussen in Brussels and Luxembourg, who grasped the possibilities inherent in the novel work emerging from these meetings, encouraged and supported the Remembering Yesterday, Caring Today project development initiated by the European Reminiscence Network. From the outset people recognised that dementia was an emerging international public health problem which transcended personal, family, national, professional, cultural and linguistic boundaries. Although a growing public issue, dementia produces considerable all too private problems for the individuals and families it affects. Remembering Yesterday, Caring Today (RYCT) evolved in the realisation that, at the individual level, reminiscence and related creative artistic activities could contribute in small but crucial ways to personal well-being, the enrichment of communication and the preservation of lifelong relationships.

Pam Schweitzer and Errollyn Bruce have been integral to the conception, evolution, development and evaluation of the RYCT approach and have personally participated in many of the separate programmes and projects based upon it throughout Europe. Here in this important manual they have distilled for all our benefits the extensive knowledge, skills and practice wisdom which they have accumulated.

I warmly commend this book to everyone concerned with needing to respond to the myriad inexorable demands which emerge in the wake of dementia. The RYCT approach seeks to preserve the humanity of people with dementing conditions. It recognises their need to have a continuing social life and to be valued for who they are. It shows family carers how they can assist this process, while at the same time having opportunities to meet and learn from other carers, thereby decreasing their own isolation, frustration and despair. It describes significant roles for volunteers and friends, who too readily evaporate when dementia sets in because they simply do not know what to do or how to help. It demonstrates to health and social care professionals and artists of many differing backgrounds the positive and pivotal actions they can take to ameliorate many of the worst social and psychological aspects emanating from dementia.

This book is hopeful, optimistic and realistic. It makes no unworkable claims and accurately presents the knowledge distilled from repeated practice. Case examples are widely used to illustrate the many practice applications, and exercises are described in detail to assist their replication. Having

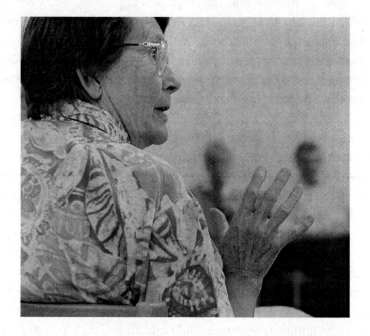

Figure F.1: Faith Gibson giving a training workshop in reminiscence in dementia care

been associated with RYCT from its earliest beginnings I am delighted to see how well the approach has blossomed in many different countries. Over the years it has evolved and developed and travelled well across national boundaries. I wholeheartedly recommend this book and the approach it advocates to people whose lives are touched in so many different ways by dementia and to those who live or work with them.

Faith Gibson,
Emeritus Professor of Social Work,
University of Ulster,
Belfast

Preface

Having long been an advocate of reminiscence work with people with dementia, it is a pleasure to welcome this volume, which presents what I believe to be an approach at the leading edge of this field. There are two key aspects that are worthy of special emphasis, and fit well with the current state of the art in dementia care. First, the RYCT approach is essentially *relationship-centred*. Involving family caregivers together with people with dementia in reminiscence sessions provides an opportunity within sessions for the relationship between the person with dementia and caregiver to be strengthened by shared memories and enhanced communication – sometimes even rediscovery of aspects of the relationship that were thought to be 'lost'. It also provides a focus for continued conversations, activity and interaction between sessions.

Second, this approach is *evidence-based*. My own first exposure to the RYCT approach was at a conference in Vienna, where the results of the first European RYCT project were being reviewed. All present were convinced of its effectiveness, although it had clearly developed slightly differently in different countries and 'hard data' on outcomes was lacking. A challenge was set down, to demonstrate rigorously that it really did have the effects that were so evident to the enthusiasts. As a result of this, Pam Schweitzer and Errollyn Bruce began to meet with Professor Martin Orrell, of University College, London, and me, to explore how evidence could be gathered that would persuade the uncommitted.

After several false starts we were successful in gaining funding from the Medical Research Council in the UK, for a trial platform, from 2004 to 2006, to prepare the ground for a definitive trial of RYCT. We were joined in this endeavour by Professor Ian Russell (like me from Bangor University), an expert on the design of trials in health and social care settings. This trial platform had several aims: one was to establish what measures would be useful to

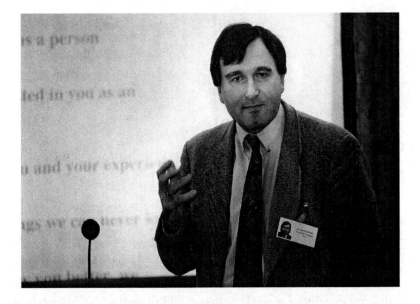

Figure P.1: Bob Woods speaking at the 1998 European Reminiscence Network conference in Vienna, which reported on the 'Remembering Yesterday, Caring Today' pilot projects conducted across Europe

evaluate the anticipated changes; another was to develop a clear, structured manual for the approach, so that it could be applied consistently, whoever was leading the groups. Pam and Errollyn had responsibility within the project for the development of the manual, and it is this which forms a core component of the current volume.

This manual is evidence based, in that it has been tried and tested in groups run in three different centres, and revised and refined accordingly. In addition, the trial platform also gave an indication, through results from 50 people with dementia and their caregivers, that this approach to reminiscence work was associated with a significant increase in autobiographical memory for people with dementia, and a significant reduction in depression for their caregivers, compared with a control group receiving no intervention. These results were sufficiently promising for the National Institute of Health Research to fund our team under their Health Technology Assessment programme to conduct a full three-year trial, involving over 500 people with dementia, expected to report in 2010. I very much hope that this book will inspire many services and organisations to explore the value of this approach in their own practice.

Bob Woods,
Professor of Clinical Psychology of Older People,
Bangor University, UK

Introduction

This book is a practical guide, containing detailed descriptions of activities for use in reminiscence groups, and ideas for one-to-one reminiscence at home or elsewhere. It is designed to give the reader a clear sense of how to use reminiscence to benefit people with dementia and those who care for them.

The major part of the book is based on ideas developed and tested over a period of ten years with people with dementia and their carers, through the 'Remembering Yesterday, Caring Today' project. This was originated and developed by the European Reminiscence Network with funding from the European Union, and ran in 16 cities across Europe. The project brought together specialists in reminiscence and in person-centred dementia care. It broke new ground by creating opportunities for people with dementia and their carers to remember together using related arts-based activities, which was, in 1997, a novel approach. The project teams in the different countries included a rich mix of psychologists, doctors, nurses, social workers, academics, poets, musicians, visual artists, theatre workers, community arts workers and oral historians. These inter-disciplinary teams brought a wealth of specialist skills and experience to the project and a fresh vision of what was possible (Schweitzer 1998).

The project, which is still running in the UK and other European countries, is aimed at families coping with dementia at home, but it can be readily adapted for use in other situations. It has been led by workers familiar with reminiscence, often with an arts background and experience of working with dementia, supported by local dementia services health workers and voluntary organisations. The emphasis is on small group activity around a different theme each week, animated by a range of multi-sensory stimuli such as objects, images, sounds and tastes to trigger memories. Stories emerging in the small groups, with support from professional group leaders, volunteers

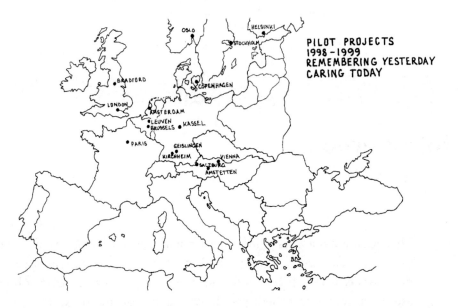

Figure I.1: European Reminiscence Network pilot projects ran in all these cities in 1997–8

and family carers, are then shared with the wider group and explored through dramatic improvisation, song, dance, drawing and writing as well as straightforward discussion. The people with dementia are given plenty of time and encouragement to enable them to participate fully in what are usually highly sociable sessions.

We have found that non-verbal exploration of memories and past skills and interests has the effect of activating and lifting the spirits of the participants and offering them ways of engaging with others, thus combating the sense of isolation and depression often associated with the experience of dementia. Such activities also remind the family carers that there are still many ways to help their relatives to communicate, even when they are finding it increasingly difficult to express themselves verbally.

In 2004 the Medical Research Council funded a preliminary study to prepare for a controlled trial of 'Remembering Yesterday, Caring Today', and for this we needed to produce a manual showing clearly how to deliver the project, so that the centres participating in the study were working to the same brief. For this, we drew upon experience of many RYCT project workers, both in the UK and in other participating countries across Europe. The manual has been tested at three different sites in the UK, both with joint groups of people with dementia and their family carers, and in groups without family carers present. It has been revised in the light of experience and evaluation. The latter half of this book brings the most up-to-date

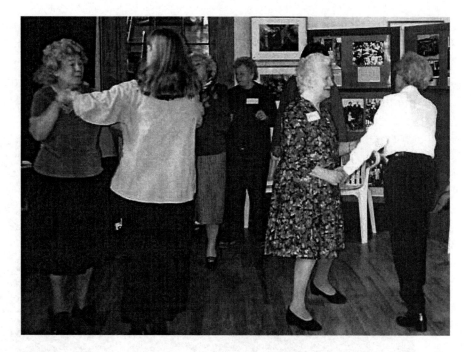

Figure I.2: Dancing days remembered in a relaxed social atmosphere

version of the manual to a wider audience. Although RYCT is a specific project, it has yielded an approach to reminiscence work with people who have dementia that can be used in many settings, and we have included advice on activities for different situations.

The book begins with an introduction to the current thinking about both reminiscence and person-centred dementia care, which came together in the development of the RYCT approach. We then consider the place and value of reminiscence in dementia care in more detail, exploring imaginative approaches to stimulating memories and reflecting on the skills required to deliver them successfully.

The following chapters offer practical advice on setting up such a reminiscence project and explore the underlying structures required to support and manage reminiscence sessions for people with dementia, with or without family carers.

Chapter 7 contains session plans for a set of themes based upon a life course framework. A range of activities is suggested for each theme, providing a ready-made planning tool for group sessions involving people with dementia and family or other carers. We also offer suggestions for ways of working in groups without family carers present and for small group or one-to-one reminiscence work. Finally we provide a range of sample documents typical of those needed to set reminiscence projects in motion.

We wish to thank all those families, project organisers, group leaders and volunteers in the centres where we have run reminiscence projects for trying out the ideas with us and giving us the benefit of their feedback.

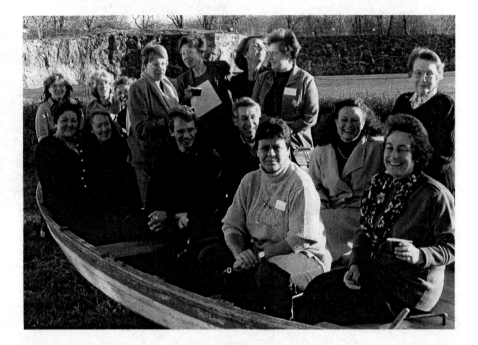

Figure I.3: European Reminiscence Network partners get together in Stockholm in 1999 to celebrate the 'Remembering Yesterday, Caring Today' pilot project's success and to plan for its future

Chapter 1

Dementia and Reminiscence

Current Thinking

DEMENTIA

As the world population ages, more and more families are coming face-to-face with dementia and adjusting their lives to cope with it. The anti-dementia drugs slow down progression for some, but they are not suitable for everybody. Research on the sedatives widely used to alleviate symptoms shows that they do very little to help, and often have unpleasant side-effects (NICE 2007). There is currently no cure for dementia, and no simple way to prevent it. This means that, for the time being, the vast majority of those who develop dementia will live with it for the rest of their lives.

The absence of a cure does not mean, however, that there is nothing we can do to help. In recent years, there has been a shift in thinking about dementia. The person-centred approach to dementia emphasises the psychological and social consequences of increasing mental frailty (Kitwood 1997). There is evidence to suggest that psychosocial interventions can significantly improve the quality of life of people with dementia and those who care for them (Brooker 2007). An important element in the person-centred approach is paying attention to what people can still do, and ways in which we can help them maintain a sense of well-being, rather than focusing mainly on their deficits and difficulties (Cheston and Bender 2000; Kitwood 1997; Sabat 2001). By creating a supportive social environment we can enable people to continue to communicate, maintain relationships and be socially included, despite their dementia.

The reminiscence approach described in this book is an example of a psychosocial intervention that is based on something we all do, and most of us enjoy – remembering and sharing stories about things we have done, places we have visited, and people who have been important to us in the past. However, if reminiscence is to be a positive experience for people with dementia, it is very important that it is done in a way that takes account of their difficulties and does not undermine them further. Taking a person-centred approach is essential to successful reminiscence work with people who have dementia.

The person-centred approach to dementia

Detailed studies of interactions between people with dementia and those who care for them have illustrated how people's relationships with others change when they have dementia. Kitwood (1997, p.4) used the phrase 'malignant social psychology' to describe the strong tendency for others to depersonalise and disempower people with dementia. His observations in care settings revealed that it is very common for the needs of people with dementia to be neglected, their feelings to be ignored or unrecognised and for them to feel marginalised and excluded in the course of their day-to-day interactions with caregivers.

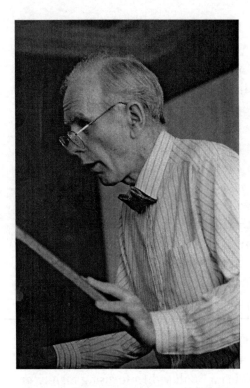

Figure 1.1: Tom Kitwood speaking at the European Reminiscence Network Conference 'Widening Horizons in Dementia Care' in 1997, which gave rise to the 'Remembering Yesterday, Caring Today' project

He referred to the different ways in which people with dementia are undermined by others as 'personal detractions'. Kitwood used strong words to describe the different types of personal detraction that he observed, but stressed that carers do not undermine people with dementia deliberately or out of malice. In his view, these ways of behaving are woven into the culture of caregiving.

Examples of personal detractions

GOING TOO FAST FOR SOMEONE (OUTPACING)
Two care workers are helping Lilian to walk from the lounge to the dining room. They are holding her arms and propelling her forwards faster than her feet can move, and she is leaning over forwards and looks very alarmed.

BEING PATRONISING (INFANTILISATION)
After helping her use the toilet, a worker says 'There's a good girl.'

USING DECEPTION (TREACHERY)
Bill keeps asking for his wife, and a worker says 'Sit down Bill, she's gone shopping and she'll be back later.' This is not true, as his wife is away, and not due back for a week.

TALKING ABOUT PEOPLE AS IF THEY WEREN'T THERE (IGNORING)
A care worker standing a few feet behind Bill's chair says to a colleague: 'Bill's been very troublesome today, going into everyone's rooms looking for his wife.'

On the positive side, Kitwood (1997) identified a number of ways in which other people can support and empower people with dementia through everyday interactions. He described this as 'positive person work' and more recently the different ways of supporting people have been termed 'personal enhancers' (Brooker and Surr 2005).

Examples of personal enhancers

CELEBRATION: RECOGNISING AND TAKING DELIGHT IN PAST AND PRESENT ACHIEVEMENTS
Lilian is very slowly eating her custard with a spoon. It keeps slipping off, but she perseveres. She is the last person sitting at the table. A care worker who is clearing other tables says 'It's nice to see you eating up your pudding. I like to see people enjoying their food.'

VALIDATION: RECOGNISING A PERSON'S REALITY, ESPECIALLY HIS OR HER EMOTIONAL REALITY
Lilian is looking for her mother. A care worker says 'Are you feeling a bit lost Lilian? I know I am not your mother, but can I do anything to help?'

WARMTH: SHOWING GENUINE CONCERN AND AFFECTION

When Bill is anxiously walking down the corridor asking for his wife, a carer takes his arm and walks with him and says, 'You must be missing Mary a lot. Let's come and find her photo, and you can tell me about her.'

INCLUDING: ENCOURAGING PEOPLE TO BE AND FEEL INCLUDED

When Bill walks into the office, the home manager says, 'Good to see you Bill. Would you like to give me a hand with something?'

The essence of person-centred care is to redress the balance in favour of supportive and positive interactions, so that people with dementia feel valued and included, though this is much easier to talk about than to put into practice.

The essential elements of person-centred care have been summed up by Brooker (2004) in the '**VIPS** framework':

1. **V**aluing people and those who care for them; promoting rights regardless of age or cognitive impairment

2. Treating people as **I**ndividuals; appreciating that each person's unique life history, personality, health status and social circumstances affect his or her experience of dementia

3. Looking at the world from the **P**erspective of each person with dementia; recognising that people are striving to make sense of their experience

4. Understanding the importance of a supportive **S**ocial environment, that provides continuing opportunities to connect and communicate with other people and feel included in a social group.

Dementia and relationships

Dementia has an enormous impact on close relationships, upsetting the established 'give and take' and causing intense feelings of loss. It can be heartbreaking to witness a partner or parent decline and change due to dementia. Family carers frequently feel ground down by the daily demands of caring, and unable to find time in the day for enjoyable activities. People with dementia tend to feel side-lined, frustrated by their difficulties and disempowered by the need to depend on others. As long-term friendships and social relationships come under strain as a result of the dementia, families often feel abandoned and experience increasing social isolation (Baldwin *et al.* 2005; Nolan, Grant and Keady 1996; Wuest, Erikson and Stern 1994). Family relationships may become stressed and it is common for the number of negative interactions between a person with dementia and family members who care for him or her to increase.

Difficult times

Bridget looked after her mother with dementia. She explained that her mother was a very independent woman, who had never liked to accept help. She was now unable to manage everyday activities like washing and dressing without assistance, but hated having help. Bridget said: 'She doesn't want anyone interfering in private matters, and she says she can manage, but of course she can't. I have to help her with washing and dressing and going to the toilet, and she hates all that. Sometimes it seems to take all day, and I get tired and cross. We used to get on well and have fun together, but now that's all gone. She won't let me help her, and says horrible things to me. I'm not a very patient person and so it gets very negative. I still love her of course, but I am not very nice to her because she is so unco-operative. I really miss her as she used to be. She's become the cuckoo in the nest, only she won't grow up and fly away, will she?'

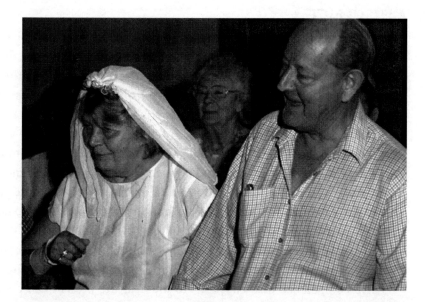

Figure 1.2: Pat and John remember their wedding day and the memory helps to bring them closer together in the present

Initially, attempts to help focused on family carers and many carer support groups were set up. More recently, the need to listen to the voices of people with dementia has been recognised (Goldsmith 1996) and support groups for them have also been organised (Yale 1999). In general, interventions working with carers and people with dementia together are a more recent development (Sheard 2004), recognising the importance of supporting the relationships between people with dementia and those who care for them at a point when they are under great pressure. The original RYCT project was an early example of working with people together for their mutual and simultaneous benefit.

Over the same period, there has been a new emphasis on the importance of relationships with paid workers (Robb *et al.* 2004). Care workers are now expected to do a great deal more than look after the basic physical needs of clients with dementia. In all health and social care settings, good communication and relationships are now seen as central to high quality care. Relationships and communication go together and depend upon understanding and respect. There is evidence that care workers who know about the life histories of their clients are more likely to empathise with them, feel warmer towards them and understand them better (Gibson 2004) and this is where reminiscence work can be so valuable.

REMINISCENCE

Reminiscence is a means of recapturing parts of the past and focusing on them to enrich our daily lives. We all do this naturally and we mostly find it enjoyable to revisit our past lives, including the recent past. Hearing other people's recollections triggers our own half-forgotten memories and can generate a collective sense of shared experience.

For older people, opportunities to talk about a shared past are often reduced by bereavement, geographical separation and physical limitations, yet the need to revisit the past and connect it with the present tends to increase with age. The desire to take stock of our lives becomes more pressing as we move towards the end of life and seek to make sense of our experience as a whole (Butler 1963; Haight and Haight 2007). One way in which older people cope with the difficulty of losing health and strength is by remembering times when they were fitter and more independent. Bringing the relative competence of their youth to mind in the present can be beneficial by putting physical ageing into perspective as just one phase in a long life.

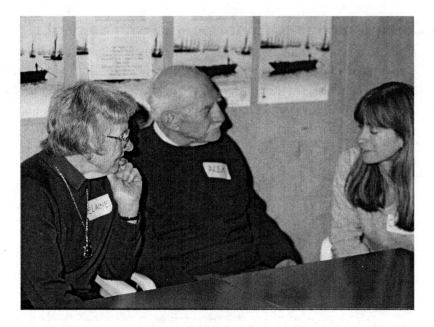

Figure 1.3: (Alex and Elaine) It can be enjoyable for couples to reminisce with an interested listener, even if the carer does most of the talking

We can meet the need to revisit the past in several ways, from responding supportively to spontaneous reminiscences, through working on a one-to-one basis, to setting up a series of structured reminiscence sessions for a group of people to pursue together. Individual work can help generate a sense of continuity between past and present and can support a person's identity. Group work adds the potential to find common ground with others, and the stimulus of a supportive 'audience'. Hearing other people's stories will often trigger long-forgotten memories, and sharing memories in a group provides a basis for new friendships.

The approach to reminiscence described here has an emphasis on the creative arts, which are used to bring stories alive in a new form, giving them a fresh focus. Using creative methods to explore and develop memories generates a sense of occasion and provides interesting ways to share and celebrate the lives of the participants. The arts are particularly appropriate for people with dementia because they give a lot of scope for non-verbal communication and emotional expression. They also provide people with dementia with opportunities to express their creativity, and to sit back and enjoy the humour and originality of other participants (Allan and Killick 2000; Bender, Bauckham and Norris 1999; Bruce, Hodgson and Schweitzer 1999; Gibson 2004; Killick and Allan 1999a and b).

Adapting reminiscence for people with dementia

Reminiscence might appear to be a surprising and inappropriate activity for people with dementia who tend to have major problems with memory, but our experience is to the contrary. Although people with dementia often have great difficulty remembering many things, they tend to have some vivid memories, particularly of events from long ago (Gibson 2004).

What is less commonly understood is that recognition is easier than recall. People with dementia often recognise stories about their own lives, and accounts of familiar times told by others, and respond with evident pleasure. Recognition persists long beyond the point where people can remember and relay their memories independently (Naess 1998).

Yes, that's quite right now you mention it

Betty, who was caring for Sybil, often told the group stories about Sybil's life as a younger woman: her skill with vehicles, her fearlessness when driving overseas, her charismatic work with children as a drama teacher, the way she cared for Betty when she was ill, which was quite often. When she spoke about Sybil, Betty would turn to her for confirmation, so that she was included in the telling, and Sybil would nod in apparent recognition and smile. Sybil could no longer speak for herself, and it is doubtful if she could remember independently, but she very much enjoyed listening in to these affirming accounts and reconnecting with her younger self.

When people with dementia recognise past times and events described by family members or by contemporaries with similar experiences, they may then spontaneously locate and contribute some of their own. There are some indications that reminiscence improves the ability of people with dementia to remember more about their own past and reconnect with their stories.

Adapting reminiscence for people with dementia involves blending good practice in reminiscence with person-centred dementia care. Because of the social and psychological consequences of dementia, we need to work in ways which enable people with dementia to participate without fear of failure. We need to recognise their real difficulties, and find ways round them by playing to their remaining strengths. We also need to take care of their feelings.

Finding ways round difficulties and playing to strengths

When doing reminiscence work with people who have dementia, the idea of playing to their strengths may seem paradoxical. People with dementia are nearly always thought to be on a downward trajectory in terms of skills and competence, but in fact many skills do remain, and may come to light when people are given sufficient encouragement and support. Maximising intact memory can enable people with dementia to surprise themselves and their carers. For example, memories of songs, both tune and words, often stay more firmly in the memory and can be called upon as a source of further memories and as a pleasurable, often communal, activity in the present.

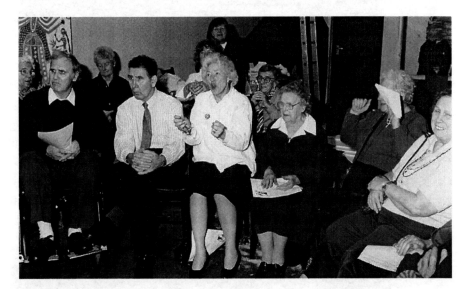

Figure 1.4: Singing remembered songs together in the London group

The body seems to have a memory, so that familiar actions relating to work, pleasure and worship are often surprisingly easy to retrieve and can provide a valuable means of communication for people with dementia in the present. For example actions connected with housework, cooking, skilled manual work, dance or sports activity can help people reconnect with an aspect of their former selves and also help them to communicate something about it to others.

People with dementia tend to be slow in marshalling their thoughts and putting them into words, so they need to be given plenty of time to respond (Sabat 2001). We must not rush in with too many prompts so that they do

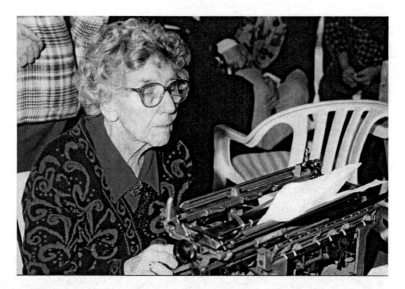

Figure 1.5: When Edith sits at the old-fashioned typewriter, she remembers immediately how to insert the paper, arrange her fingers for typing and make the carriage-return work with a satisfying ring

not know what to respond to first. They should not feel under pressure to speak, but we should not assume that they do not want to. Because it is hard to predict when someone will suddenly be prompted to contribute, we should always offer the chance and ensure that wherever possible there is a worker or volunteer available to listen if the moment to speak arises.

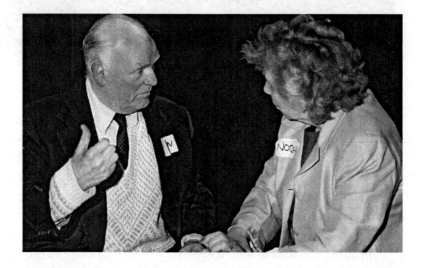

Figure 1.6: Nora, a volunteer, talks with Martin, allowing time for him to gather his thoughts and listening attentively

In recent years there has been a great deal of work in the dementia care field exploring what we need to do to have successful conversations with people who have dementia. Our own feelings are crucial. We must approach conversations with people who have dementia convinced that they have something to say, or there is a great risk that our body language will convey that we do not expect much response and are not really interested. There are also a number of relatively simple techniques that we can use to enable people with dementia to express themselves (Killick and Allan 2001; Powell 2000; Sabat 2001).

Examples of ways to enable people with dementia in conversation

- When we keep our own turns brief and allow the people with dementia plenty of time to gather their thoughts and express themselves, we are signalling that we are prepared to listen and value their contribution.

- Tolerating silences and avoiding the temptation to fill them by saying something yourself. When we fill silences, we risk interrupting a person's attempts to formulate his or her thoughts. We need to allow that person extra time to enable him or her to speak – pauses of ten seconds may feel awkward at first, but may be all it takes to give a person time to say something. People with severe dementia may speak if you listen attentively for longer periods, for example ten minutes, and this is something that can be tried when doing one-to-one work.

- Repeating back to people what they have said so far, when sentences suddenly dry up after a confident beginning. Saying 'You were just telling me about the time when…' or 'We were talking about friends and you were mentioning your friend from next door…'. This will sometimes help the person to go back and carry on with the story.

- Keeping the point of view of people with dementia in mind. We can use our understanding of their feelings and their perceptions of the world to help make sense of what they are saying if it is not entirely clear.

- Providing a missing word if they are struggling to find one, but then allowing them to carry on.

- Checking our understanding by restating what we think they are saying, and asking them to say if we have got it right – for example 'Let me see if I understand, you are saying that...'.

- Offering help very tactfully. Psychologically, there is a huge difference between a listener who points out and corrects mistakes (correcting the speaker) and one who checks out whether he or she has grasped what the speaker is saying correctly (checking the listener's understanding).

We can also explore non-verbal means of communication (Perrin and May 2000). For example, when we invite people to 'show us how it was', we can often liberate the tongue-tied story-teller, who may be well able to demonstrate how something was done, but cannot put it into words.

Replaying the washboard

Given a washboard, a block of soap and an old shirt, Lily demonstrated a past washday and behaved as though it was happening now in the present, yet when we had asked her earlier in the session how washing was done, she did not seem to remember and could not tell us anything about it.

By using as many senses as possible, we can bypass difficulties with words and give people maximum chance of receiving an idea and responding to it. Using familiar objects from the past as memory prompts can help with recall, as the hand feels the weight of an object, its texture, the eye sees its shape and the body replays associated movements.

Images too, whether of family members and personal events or of local scenes or significant public events, can stimulate memories and conversation, especially if enlarged in size, making all important details easy to see. Drawing and painting can also help some people to express their past when words do not come easily (Chaudhury 2003).

Being part of a re-enactment of a familiar situation puts people in a position to participate in a group activity without feeling under pressure, and to show through their actions that they understand.

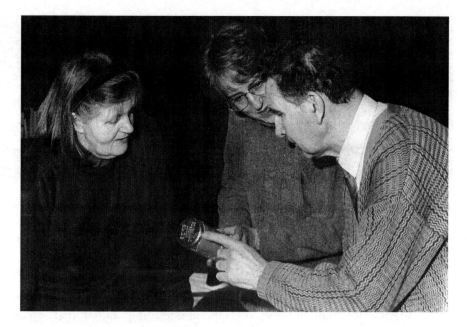

Figure 1.7: James finds an object which triggers memories to share

Back to school

Taking part in a re-enactment of a school day gave plenty of opportunities for participation without risk of exposure. The group leader took the role of the teacher with a blackboard and chalk to stimulate memories and props were placed around the room, such as a globe, a cane, slates, a pencil box and a ruler. The seats were arranged in rows and the whole group of people with dementia, carers and volunteers stood and sat on command. They chanted times tables and sang familiar hymns as though in school. This allowed people with dementia to join in where they could and to feel part of the activity, including appreciating the pranks of fellow-pupils!

The art of remembering

Lesley found it very difficult to speak, but he had always enjoyed drawing and retained his skill in this area. He sat quietly looking at an old wood planing tool which clearly reminded him of one he had used himself. He then drew it very carefully and was fully absorbed in this activity. He was gratified by the praise his artwork produced from the rest of the group when the drawing was passed round.

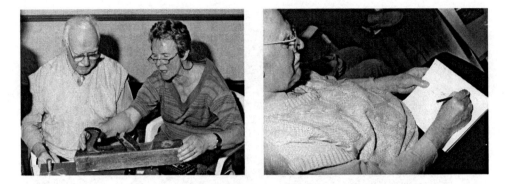

Figures 1.8a and b: Leslie and Maggie explore the old wooden box plane together and then Leslie draws it

Taking care of feelings

People with dementia tend to feel very vulnerable because their daily experience is that they are constantly getting things wrong, and others frequently respond to them in ways that are undermining rather than enhancing (Brooker 2007). When doing reminiscence work, we want them to feel that they have made a valuable contribution whenever they offer a response, be it an action, a word or a sentence. Recognising that everything they contribute represents an achievement and obstacles overcome, we must be careful to acknowledge that and not to correct people when what they say or do seems unlikely. When they make an appropriate response, however small, we need to give them a great deal of praise and appreciation. We can amplify their comments by repeating them back and linking them with the overall content and flow of the session. In this way, we can help people with dementia to stay at the heart of the process and not to feel marginalised or excluded.

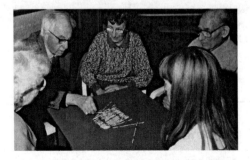

Figure 1.9: Concentrating on a game of Pick-up-Sticks in a group session on childhood games

The more imaginative we become in finding ways of engaging and actively involving people with dementia in activities where they can succeed, the longer we can help them maintain their confidence, sense of self and motivation to communicate. In later chapters we discuss in greater detail different ways to stimulate memories.

Chapter 2

Reminiscence in Dementia Care

REASONS FOR USING REMINISCENCE IN DEMENTIA CARE

To get to know and understand people better

If we are aiming to provide person-centred care, we need to know and understand the people we care for. Bell and Troxel (2001) have argued that life history is as important to holistic care as medical history is to medical care. People with dementia have lived long lives and, to understand them as they are now, we need to know as much as possible about them and the times they have lived through. We may have some basic information about their life history through their case notes, but we can find out much more about people when we show an interest in their past, encourage them to tell their own stories and take note of what they say.

Telling a story about the past involves recreating it each time it is told, which means that it differs according to the mood of the teller and who is listening. This can be confusing, since there can often seem to be little connection between two tellings of 'the same' story, but it does not necessarily point to confusion or inaccuracy on the part of the teller, whether or not that person has dementia. So whatever others may feel about apparent inaccuracies, we should assume that what a person chooses to communicate about his or her past life has the potential to tell us something, both about that life, and about how the person is feeling in the present.

Pause for thought

You will almost certainly understand what we are saying if you think about your own experience as a listener, and teller, of stories.

- Is the telling of the story of an incident during a wild night out different as told to parents, friends or the police?

- Do you know someone who talks of her marriage (job, childhood, etc.) as a total disaster when she is depressed, but accepts that it has ups and downs when she is feeling happy?

- Do you have things in your own life that you talk about differently depending on your mood and who you are with?

People with dementia (and those without) often tell us things we have heard before, and it is tempting to switch off (Bruce 1998). However, if we decide to listen and pay attention to the way the story is told, asking supplementary questions to show we are listening and are interested, we may find that we get to know new things about them, even from an oft-repeated story, and that we can be clearer about why they tell it so often (Knocker 2002).

Reminiscence as a means of promoting conversation and communication

For many people, the onset of dementia and the communication difficulties it can bring involves the loss of enjoyable conversation, especially the on-going conversations of a lifetime with close family and friends. Cognitive losses mean that it becomes more difficult to formulate coherent thoughts, and loss of language makes it hard to express thoughts in words. The fear of making mistakes may discourage people from attempting to communicate, and the tendency for other people to show little interest in what they have to say, and to fail to make allowances for their difficulties in saying it, creates additional barriers.

In care homes there are many opportunities for conversation with people with dementia, but they are not always maximised. Studies suggest that carers' conversations with people who have dementia tend to be very brief; frequently there is very little conversation during personal care tasks (Ward *et al.* 2005) and often the interaction that takes place is not very satisfactory for the person with dementia (Hallbierg *et al.* 1995). Some family carers may report that there is 'no conversation' and this may come about because living with dementia changes the nature of family relationships so much. Family members often find it hard to manage without the easy verbal communication they had in the past, and find it difficult to accept changes and be content with different, and usually reduced, channels of communication. However, through participation in a reminiscence group, they can learn by example and from one another how to trigger memories in a variety of different ways and be rewarded with smiles of recognition, and sometimes with a recollection they have never heard before.

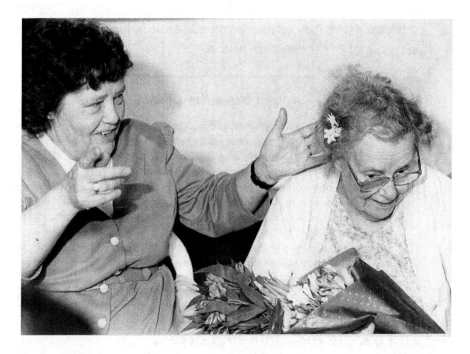

Figure 2.1: May and her daughter Pat celebrating May's 100th birthday with the reminiscence group

Recapturing the fun

A daughter and her mother participated in a reminiscence group together. The daughter commented that it had made her realise that for a long time she and her mother had only been talking about lost money, lost keys and a host of worries and problems. Through going to the group together they learned to leave practical things behind and have much more fun together, looking at old photos and remembering happy times, at home as well as in the meetings.

Reminiscence as a confidence-building activity

When people talk about and re-enact their earlier lives, they can sometimes get back in touch with competence and energy associated with earlier times. Some of this energy then spills over into the present day, so that they probably feel, and certainly seem, younger and more confident. For example, when a group of older women talk together about memories of dressing up to go out dancing, the excitement and glamour of the remembered occasion infuses the way they describe it, giving them and the listener a sense of them as energetic, attractive and socially competent young women. This renewed connection with their youth is positive and also helps others present to get a keener sense of the complete person.

May I have the pleasure?

A group of people with dementia and their carers were taking part in a session on dancing days. They were arranged up two opposite sides of the wall, as was often the case in dance halls of old. The 'boys and girls' were winking at members of the opposite sex and making non-verbal contact, deciding who they would, and would not, like to dance with. When the 'wrong' boy asked her to dance, one of the ladies used the tactic she remembered from her youth: 'Sorry, I'm with my friend,' but when a more attractive partner came along, she nudged her partner and said, 'This one's OK!' and got up to dance. Like many people with dementia, her comic timing had not disappeared and she was able to make everyone laugh.

Helping people maintain and access autobiographical memory

People with dementia lose access to significant amounts of memory, and this includes both recent memories and those from the past. Typically, however, there are some memories from the distant past which are well preserved and opportunities to share these memories may help to conserve them longer. Reminiscence can also reactivate long-lost memories in a way which is surprising and delightful for the person and for those who have helped this to happen. Very often these memories resurface spontaneously when sensory stimulus or input from other people touches a nerve (Gibson 2004). For example, the feel of a silk stocking slipped on to the arm can evoke memories of a special day long ago, or the mention of a particular cinema or dance hall by someone else triggers a set of memories related to that place.

If dementia progresses and memories fade irretrievably, there is great comfort for the person in hearing his or her story relayed, provided the telling (whether by a relative or carer) is reasonably accurate and sensitive. As mentioned in the previous chapter, many people with dementia recognise their stories when they hear them, even though they can no longer tell them themselves, and keeping their stories alive is a way of helping them hold on to their sense of self.

Keeping conversation going

Don's wife complained bitterly that he never talked to her any more. She missed the conversations they used to have about goings-on in the family, the village, and the world at large. But Don's son Jeff discovered that he could keep conversation going with his father by getting him talking about the past. Don had been a great raconteur, and Jeff remembered many of the stories he told about amusing incidents from his time as a travelling salesman. Jeff said 'As he got worse, he'd forget what his old stories were, but I remembered them, and I could tell them to him, and then he'd remember, you know. He'd perk up and find something to say.'

Developing group belonging

In many care settings the need for care is the only reason why people find themselves together. They often feel misplaced in a group of strangers with whom they have nothing in common. Group reminiscence can bring out common experiences and foster relationships. For example, it may emerge through discussion that group members worked in the same trade or attended the same school, church or dance hall.

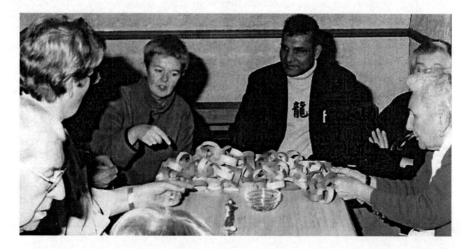

Figure 2.2: Christmas memories are shared while working together on paper chains to decorate the room

The sense of being part of a valued social group is greatly enhanced by participating in an enactment together. This can be set up quite simply by slightly rearranging the room and declaring it to be somewhere else: for example, a schoolroom (with chairs set out in rows), a dance hall with chairs up both sides (for young men and women to give each other the eye!), a church on the occasion of a wedding with chairs arranged as pews, or a charabanc with chairs in twos all facing one way (Schweitzer 2007).

It takes a bit of courage to disturb the furniture, but the resulting increase in energy and imagination makes it worthwhile and rewarding. It is easier for people with dementia to participate in a session on memories of going to the seaside, for example, if the chairs are arranged in pairs and rows like a coach and they are sitting next to a volunteer or worker on this 'coach'. Using imaginary prompts, such as the beginnings of the countryside, seagulls wheeling overhead and the first sight of the sea, they can increase the engagement of the person with dementia and find out more about where he or she liked to go for holidays or daytrips. And recreating the sort of classroom which most people will be familiar with can enable people with dementia to participate confidently just by joining in where they can, without having to risk solo story-telling.

Form an orderly queue please

In a session on cinemas, we arranged the chairs in rows facing a blank wall, 'the screen'. The whole group (people with dementia, carers, volunteers and staff) formed a queue to go in, except for Ted, a volunteer, who was the commissionaire, with a peaked cap to prove it! Ted made them form an orderly line (which of course they didn't) and Nora started to sing a song remembered from childhood about being 'Members of the ABC', which was a chain of cinemas at the time. Lots of people knew this song and joined in while they were in 'the queue'. The commissionaire let them in one at a time and they filled up the cinema seats. Olive, the pianist (an older volunteer), played classic themes from different kinds of films (horror, slap-stick, romance) and 'the audience' responded as though they were really watching such films, pointing up at the imaginary screen, covering their eyes with fear, swooning in the romantic bits, etc. At the end, Olive played 'God save the King' and they all stood up, some of them shuffling back into imaginary tight shoes or edging along the rows to get out quickly for the last bus! Luckily we filmed this session, so we were able to relive the fun of it all the following week, appreciating one another's creativity, and enjoying a feeling that we were a really good group to belong to.

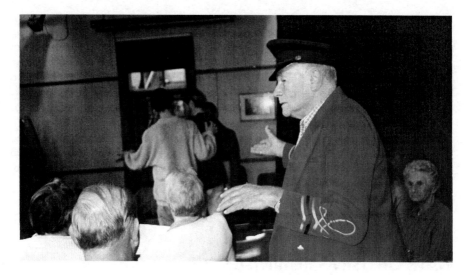

Figure 2.3: Ted, a volunteer, as commissionaire shows people to their cinema seats

Celebrating difference

Reminiscence work is also a good way to celebrate differences and help people with different backgrounds to feel included and valued in a group. In the right atmosphere it can be exciting to hear about experiences which are different from one's own (Bender *et al.* 1999; Schweitzer 2004). For example, it can be very stimulating for the whole group to hear about going through a very different school system in another country or about how weddings are conducted in another culture, or how the changing seasons of the year are marked with special festivals. It can provide a good way to acknowledge the positive side of diversity, though it is always important to be on the look out for negative labels based on differences.

Season of mists and mellow fruitfulness
(notes on an autumn session)

We used as many whole-group activities as possible in this session, with everyone joining in. We started with a brainstorm on words and situations connected with autumn. Things like mist and fog were mentioned, hop-picking, conkers, autumn leaves, getting dark early and back to school. There were also stories from Japan (from Noriko, a student working with us) about Japanese autumn rituals, and from Mr Malik we heard about what happens at Ramadan.

Jean mentioned that there was often fog on the local heath in the early autumn mornings and the whole group moved from one side of the room to the other, pretending not to be able to see where they were going, banging into each other and apologising. We all joined in Margaret's memories of hop-picking by pretending to be collecting hops off the vine and putting them in a big communal hop-bin. Betty remembered a few lines of Keats's 'Ode to Autumn' and we tried to piece it together (unsuccessfully) in the group… (Note: I must remember to look for the poem and take it in next week!) Noriko taught us a Japanese song about the autumn, holding up a big collage based on her own memories with an arrangement of autumn leaves and painted fires. And Mr Malik told us about what it was like to fast during Ramadan. I had the feeling that we all felt part of the global village and enjoyed hearing about how autumn feels in other countries, both similarities and differences.

WAYS OF USING REMINISCENCE IN DEMENTIA CARE

In this section we will discuss some of the ways in which reminiscence can contribute to delivering person-centred care in care homes, day care centres and community settings catering for people with dementia (Bruce and Schweitzer 2008). However, most of the ideas can also be used by family carers or practitioners supporting people with dementia living at home.

Using reminiscence when gathering information about life history

Knowledge of life history can help dementia caregivers in many ways such as:

- understanding what people are saying, when their speech is not clear

- decoding the messages in baffling behaviour

- appreciating people's preferences and tastes and accommodating them as far as possible

- understanding habits and routines which relate to the past but are evident in present behaviour.

Much can be found out about a person's life by asking family carers and they can provide good 'factual' information. However, we also need to hear and value people's own version of their stories, told in their own way. Getting the facts right is not everything; reminiscence work recognises the importance of the emotional truth expressed in the telling of the story.

Where people are committed to providing high quality care for people with dementia, there is a growing interest in finding out about life history, and finding ways to improve the recording of information. Patchy biographical notes hidden away in a filing cabinet are not very helpful. Caregivers need to have constant and easy access to life story material to retain a real sense of who they are caring for and how they have lived the earlier parts of their lives. Sometimes it is small details that explain current behaviour (Bell and Troxel 1997; Kitwood 1997). Reminiscence, along with information provided by families, can be a way to find out more.

Alone in bed for the first time

John Style moved to a nursing home when his wife died from a heart attack. He was very distressed by this double loss of his wife and of his home and familiar surroundings. As the months went on he became less distressed and began to settle down, clearly enjoying company. However he was very restless at night, constantly waking up and coming to look for the night staff. He was always reluctant to go back to bed. At this time, his key worker Karen was gathering information about John's life. She spent some time with John talking about his memories. John told her a lot about his twin brother and four sisters, a big family in a small house. When Karen asked him if he shared a room with his brother, he said 'not just a room, shared a bed, right up till I married.'

Karen realised that John had never slept alone until he moved into the nursing home at the age of 85. She suspected that this might explain his restlessness and suggested that the night staff experimented with various things such as going into his room and touching John when doing their checks, using a night light, leaving the radio on low. While it was never entirely clear which of these things made a difference, night staff felt that understanding how John might be feeling made things easier for them, and over time he did wake less often, and return to bed more willingly.

Reminiscence 'on the hoof' during routine caregiving

We have already mentioned that having dementia puts communication and conversation at risk. This is not just the result of difficulties with memory, thinking, speech and language. It is also because caregivers do not always give the encouragement and help that people with dementia need, and indeed, may unwittingly do the reverse, as we indicated earlier.

When conversation becomes rare, people with dementia can feel isolated and alone, even when they are surrounded by other people. Their need for care means that they are receiving help from caregivers at regular intervals, and this provides an ideal opportunity for conversation. In care settings with a commitment to person-centred care and an emphasis on communication, staff make good use of reminiscence as a vehicle to stimulate conversation (Bell and Troxel 1997). With activities of daily living – such as dressing, bathing, brushing hair, snuggling down in bed – the physical experience of the action involved can trigger memories. If care is delivered sensitively, the intimate nature of these activities provides a moment conducive to sharing thoughts and feelings. However, these moments are lost if tasks are seen as something to get over and done with as quickly as possible.

Grasping the moment

As Carol (care worker) was washing Mabel's back with a soapy sponge, she said 'My mum used to do that.' It was rare for Mabel to say so much, and Carol replied by saying 'Sounds like a lovely mum' and waited for a few moments to see if Mabel would say more. After a long pause, Mabel said 'She's waiting for me…won't be long now.' Sensing that Mabel was saying something important, but not sure how to take it, Carol stopped washing Mabel and looked at her intently while thinking what to say. Eventually she said: 'And you're a lovely daughter to be waiting for.' She then got on with the task of helping Mabel out of the bath. Ten days later, when Mabel had a stroke and never regained consciousness, Carol was relieved that she had taken a bit of extra time to connect with Mabel that day.

Carers can use the physical actions of the moment to invite memories of how these activities were done by parents and grandparents, or perhaps by the people themselves as young parents. There are many memories attached to washing, bathing and choosing clothes, and with a little encouragement many people with dementia will have something to say about, for example, what they wore as a child, who chose their clothes and whether they liked them or not.

As we have already suggested, life stories need to come out of the filing cabinet if they are to be accessible to staff (Gibson 2004). It is helpful to have immediate prompts available on the walls or on shelves in the places where care is being delivered to help stimulate conversation and to remind carers that the people on the receiving end of their caregiving are individuals with their own histories and long lives behind them. A set of photographs with captions mounted on the wall, some records of past achievements, mementos, a life story collage or a memory box – all of these will act as aide-memoires for the person with dementia and as a source of ideas for conversation and communication for the carer.

Display boards

A French care home had a display board in each room presenting important details about the residents' lives. There were names and photos of close family and friends, favourite pets and other important elements in each person's life, for example places where they had lived, worked or gone on holiday. Carers could initiate conversation by commenting on something on the board, and found that it was much easier to respond appropriately when residents talked about their past lives. If, for example, a resident began to talk about Jacques they could glance at the board, to see whether Jacques was a brother, husband, son or a dog.

Creating a stimulating environment

The display boards in the French care home are a simple way to use the environment to encourage communication and conversation. A great deal can be done to make the environments in which people with dementia spend their time more stimulating. Some care settings have experimented with creating an environment rich in pictures and objects likely to stimulate the senses and trigger memories.

Corridors with a focus

In Copenhagen some care homes and other meeting places for older people now have lively reminiscence corners and stopping points in their corridors. These areas, created by the Danish Reminiscence Centre, are decorated with small murals, objects and photos focusing on themes known to be of interest to some of the residents, such as fishing or enjoying the great outdoors.

People's own homes have many things about the place connected with their activities and interests, and these are often cleared away when people become old and frail, or lost when they move into care. When carers become aware of the value of such prompts, they think more carefully before dispensing with them.

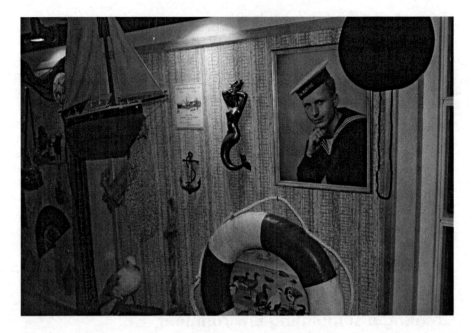

Figure 2.4: Ove Dahl, founder of the Danish Reminiscence Centre, created special interest corners to stimulate discussion, such as this nautical themed display

---

Reminiscence trail at home

Inge's mother used to walk from room to room a great deal. Inge had the idea of creating a reminiscence trail so that her mother had something interesting and stimulating to discover as she walked around the house. For example, on the hall table she put a pair of leather driving gloves, an old map of the local area, a visiting card and an old hat. Above the table were some photos of the family on various outings. In each room in the house there was a small collection of memorable objects for her mother to handle and photos to prompt memories. Inge said that her mother still walked a lot, but seemed less anxious and restless.

Providing objects to handle gives people an opportunity to occupy themselves pleasurably and this has been tried successfully on quite an ambitious scale by putting an old car in the garden for people to sit in, polish or tinker with, or providing a potting shed or greenhouse, with a selection of pots, compost and tools that people can use safely.

Many care homes encourage families to personalise rooms, and some have display cabinets outside, or a place to put a photo that will help people recognise their own rooms. A Norwegian home used recent photos, but when one resident asked about the 'old lady' on her door, they discovered

---

Special activity corners to visit

The New Horizons homes have corners in the main living area associated with particular aspects of life such as a mirror with jewellery and make-up, a sewing corner, a work/office corner and a childhood memories corner with toys and dolls to handle as residents please and boys' and girls' annuals from the past.

---

that many people preferred, and were better able to recognise, a photo of themselves when they were young. This was not a denial of age or a nostalgic retreat into the past, but rather a recognition of how people view themselves and their lives, and it helped to create an environment that was meaningful to the residents.

Reminiscence as a group activity

Reminiscence can be done as an activity with individuals or in groups, with varying amounts of input from family members in each case. This work can be done within care settings (such as day centres and homes), in the community or at home.

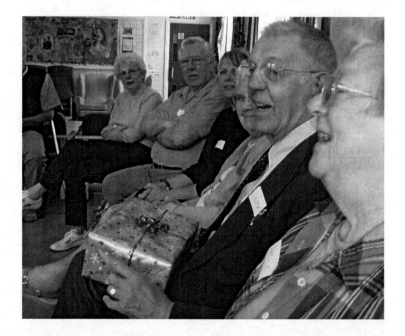

Figure 2.5: A Christmas memories session in Bradford where Charlie tells about a favourite present in a game of Pass the Parcel

Reminiscence group work is probably the most common reminiscence activity used with people who have dementia. Many care homes report that they are doing reminiscence work (DSDC Wales 2002). However, it is important to be reflective about the quality of this work, and aware of what is needed to make it worthwhile. After such a session, it is good practice to think through what happened, how the individuals involved reacted and what can be improved.

One-off reminiscence sessions can be organised to mark a special occasion, a seasonal event, a festival or a Christmas party. Family carers may well be willing to assist with preparations and to participate in the session and this can give them a sense of the potential of reminiscence as a source of conversation. Community groups may want to organise occasional reminiscence sessions as part of their programme.

A one-off session

A one-off reminiscence session was scheduled at an Alzheimer's café in July. The group had chosen 'summer holidays and trips' as the theme for the session. The venue was normally set up like a café, with small groups sitting at round tables. For the reminiscence session tables and chairs were arranged so that people could easily move from working in small groups to being in a large circle with a space in the middle. This was ideal for enactments based on people's memories. Everyone had a chance to join in with the Sunday School picnic (opening imaginary packs of sandwiches in brown paper and saying what was in them), be a passenger on a coach trip (chairs arranged in pairs, and one pair behind another), play games on the beach or take part in a dramatic sea fishing trip (a visualisation of the waves churning and actions of pulling in the fish). Sandwiches and ice cream added to the normal refreshments. As she was leaving, one participant said, 'Thank you so much, I've had a lovely day out.'

Reminiscence can be a good way to celebrate a personal event such as someone's birthday or anniversary. In collaboration with family and friends, there can be a 'This is Your Life' session for the individual or couple, to which they listen and participate when they feel like it. The experience of being celebrated by others in the room, with stories supported by photos or perhaps film footage, gives a sense of pride and value to the person and brings something special to the occasion. It is also a good way to mark the passing of a life.

You will find advice on good practice and ideas for activities you can use in reminiscence group work in Chapters 3–7.

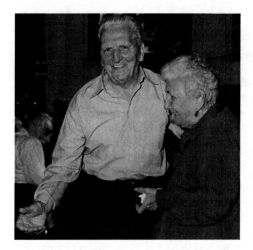

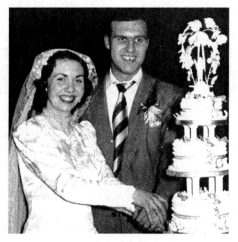

Figure 2.6: Bob and Doll celebrate their wedding anniversary with the memories group

Figure 2.7: This wedding photo brought in from home by Dennis and Nora of their special day brought many memories and much remembered happiness for the couple

---

This is Your Life

At her mother's funeral Stella put photos on display boards and told the story of her mother's life, picking out memorable events and details that illustrated her mother's personality and talents. When the funeral was over she commented 'Mum would have loved to have heard that. What a pity I left it until her funeral. And it would have been nice for the staff in her nursing home to have heard it while they were still looking after her.'

Reminiscence as a one-to-one activity

If you are working in a setting where serious attempts are made to find appropriate activities for everyone (Brooker and Woolley 2007), individual reminiscence sessions can be a good way to work with people who do not readily join in with group activities. As mentioned, one-to-one sessions can be used when collecting life history information and they lie at the heart of structured life review (Haight and Haight 2007). They may also be valuable as a means of gathering clues helpful to understanding present anxiety or distress. The stories remembered may give a clue as to what is upsetting somebody and in any case the personal attention involved in listening and being with the person may be just what is needed.

Helping to cope with distress through positive reminiscence

Lise Naess in Norway worked with individuals using a mixture of basic information, guesswork and background knowledge of the times to explore the memories and feelings of people with dementia. When an elderly man frequently tried to leave the home saying he must go to his mother, she started talking to him about his mother and their relationship in his childhood. 'Ah, I am sure your mother was a lovely mum when you were little? I bet she cooked good meatballs. And I expect she picked you up when you fell and hurt yourself. Have you a photo of your mother in your room?' Together they went to his room to look at a photo of his mother and she reminded him that he had looked after his mother when she got older and he was grown up. He then remembered that his mother was dead. After several repeats of this one-to-one activity, when the man wanted his mother, he would agree to look at her photo rather than insist that he must leave the home.

One-to-one reminiscence work can fruitfully involve family members, and is an especially valuable way to work with people who are still living at home.

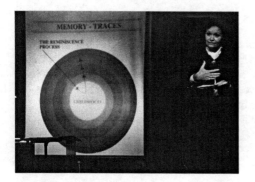

One-to-one sessions benefit from being structured and planned (perhaps chronologically or around different life themes) so that appropriate triggers can be located for each session and there is a greater sense of purpose. It is important to let the person have a say in the agenda, and be prepared to change the plan if he or she is reluctant to explore a chosen theme.

If a person has problems with speech and language, we need to take a creative approach to communication and to make full use of non-verbal clues (Killick and Allan 2001). For example, we can observe closely for signs that might indicate whether a chosen topic has any appeal. If there are positive signs and we feel that there is mileage in the subject, we need to explore it in ways which do not require extensive speech on that person's part, but instead a yes/no answer or a physical response.

Figure 2.8: Lise Naess, clinical psychologist from Norway, speaks about accessing long-term memory at a European Reminiscence Network conference on dementia in London

It is also possible to work collaboratively on drawing a memory, working within the person's limitations. In this case the worker can use guesswork and available knowledge to start drawing and ask for feedback, which can be nodding and shaking the head or thumbs up and down.

Drawing the teacher

In a one-to-one session on the theme of schooldays, a carer tried to find out about a man's memories of his teachers – loved or hated. She started drawing, asking questions all the time, such as 'Is it a man or a woman?', 'Shall we give him a cane, or perhaps a ruler?' or 'What did he wear? Did he have glasses?', 'Should he be smiling or frowning in the picture?', 'Did he ever punish you?' or 'Did he ever give you a special prize?' As the information was retrieved, the details were added to the picture, which was by no means a work of art, but rather a jointly created record of his memories. He took the picture home and it sparked a discussion with his family.

Similarly one can use short enactments of stories from the person's life, guessing how parts of conversations might have gone, amending them in the light of the person's suggestions, and looking for ways to use humour and character to bring the remembered situation to life again for the person.

Acting up

A worker took on the role of a young girl who wanted the money to go to the cinema and she asked the person with dementia to play her mother. The 'daughter' mentioned a well-known film from the period of the person's youth and said it was on at the local cinema of those days, the Splendid. She asked for the money to go. The 'mother' said: 'I gave you money last week.' 'Oh please Mum,' wheedled the 'daughter', 'I'll be good and I'll do the shopping for you.' Back came the reply from the person in role as mother: 'You'll have to ask your father.' She was delighted to join in the enactment which gave her a chance to be funny and to show understanding of this archetypal situation.

Process and product

Working towards a tangible result can provide a focus for reminiscence work and make it more meaningful to the person you are working with. The advantage of making a product, if it is attractively produced, is that it is something to be proud of, both for the maker and for the person whose memories are illustrated.

At its simplest, this can involve typing up a person's memory as told in a recent session, printing it out and enlarging it to put on the wall. This can serve as an aide-memoire to an earlier part of life and it can also remind the person of an enjoyable recent reminiscence experience, as well as providing a useful conversation stimulus for staff and visitors.

REMINISCENCE AND DEMENTIA – A NOTE ON THE EVIDENCE BASE

Reminiscence has been used in many different ways, and reminiscence projects have a wide variety of aims and objectives. Like other psychosocial interventions, reminiscence work has many elements, and it is not easy to separate them and say which is responsible for its impact. Reminiscence work is not expected to have the same effects on everyone – there are a range of possible benefits, and it is at its best when tailored to individual needs. This presents a challenge when using quantitative research methods designed to investigate standard treatments that are expected to affect everyone in much the same way. The current Cochrane review of reminiscence therapy (Woods et al. 2005) illustrates this inherent difficulty, as only four trials suitable for analysis were found, each evaluating different kinds of reminiscence work.

Evidence from other kinds of research, and from experience, suggests that working with life history can be very valuable to care workers, family members and people with dementia themselves (Bender et al. 1999; Gibson 2004). A review of research on group reminiscence for people with dementia suggested that the main positive outcomes reported were increased levels of engagement, enjoyment and communication (Woods and McKiernan 1995). More recently, a study using Dementia Care Mapping found greater levels of well-being in participants during reminiscence than in other types of group activity for people with dementia in day care settings (Brooker and Duce 2000). Gibson (2004) has emphasised the importance of the effects of reminiscence work on caregivers – something that has seldom been the main focus of research. When reminiscence work softens negative attitudes and improves the quality of relationships between people with dementia and those who care for them, there are significant implications for quality of care.

A recent review of life story work in dementia care (Moos and Bjorn 2006) concludes that we still have a great deal to learn about how best to use life stories in the delivery of sensitive, individualised and effective support and care to people with dementia, and warns against rushing into rigorous quantitative studies prematurely. Woods (2003) argued that we need to foster the development of creative approaches to reminiscence and allow time for them to be piloted and refined before undertaking controlled trials. He also suggested that the outcome measures used in trials need to reflect the type of reminiscence work and its aims (Woods 2002).

For practitioners examining their own practice, Cohen-Mansfield (2005) suggests key questions are: Will this intervention suit particular clients? If so, how can we tailor it to meet their needs? What do we need to do to maximise the chances that it will be beneficial? To answer these questions, evidence from qualitative studies and experience is invaluable, and the practical suggestions in this book are largely based on evidence of this kind.

As Bob Woods explains in the preface, the Remembering Yesterday, Caring Today programme is to be evaluated in a multi-centre randomised controlled trial. This research will evaluate the programme looking at a small number of specific outcomes for people with dementia and their carers, and its cost effectiveness. It will provide the kind of evidence favoured by commissioners and policy makers responsible for funding and coordinating services.

Chapter 3

Reminiscence Skills and Methods

ATTITUDES AND SKILLS NEEDED FOR SUCCESSFUL REMINISCENCE WORK

> Attitudes, values, knowledge and skills are more important than any particular professional background. Skills can be learned... (Gibson 1998, p.18)

Some of the essential skills listed below may sound so obvious that they do not need pointing out. It is true that some people are 'naturals' when it comes to engaging with older people and valuing their memories, but the majority of us need to put some thought into developing our skills.

- **Good listening skills**: be very attentive to what each speaker is saying, showing that you are 'there' for them, and do not rush to prompt or question. People with dementia often need extra time in order to formulate and express their thoughts so be prepared to wait in silence for their response.

- **Receptiveness**: relax, and show in your body language, including eye contact, that you are pleased to be listening and that you are interested and value what is being said.

- **Curiosity**: you need to have a genuine desire to know more and to learn from the older people, especially as they will be very quick to stop reminiscing if they feel you are bored or doing this work out of duty.

- **Sensitivity**: make yourself receptive to the feelings which the speaker is revealing, as well as the content, especially where a painful memory may have been triggered, and guard against questioning which may be experienced as intrusive.

- **An accepting attitude**: do not judge the person remembering, but rather show that you have heard and understood what he or she said and respect his or her point of view.

- **A reasonable memory**: you must be able to recall what has been said and be able to refer back to it, in order to make the person remembering feel it is worthwhile talking to you, and so you can make links between different stories he or she has told.

- **A sense of humour**: you need to be able to create an easy atmosphere, sharing the funny side of things remembered, and delighting in the unexpected and bizarre.

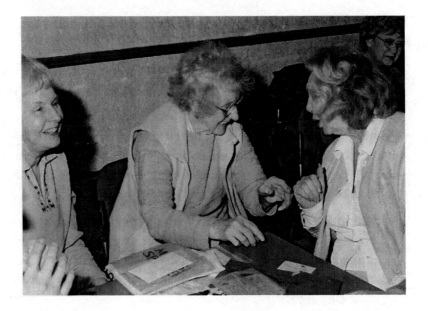

Figure 3.1: Pleasurable conversation and fun in a small group: mother and daughter and Nora, an experienced volunteer in London

- **Adaptability**: you must be willing to change plans quickly and 'go with' the interests and needs of the person. What is important is that the person has a chance to communicate immediately what he or she wants to say, rather than having to stick with a specific chosen topic.

- **Co-operative conversational strategies**: try speaking at a pace which matches that of the person, leaving pauses which mirror his or her own. Do not be tempted to fill the gaps too quickly. If you are not sure you have understood what someone is saying, then you can reflect back what you think you have heard with words like: 'Have I got this right?' (Sabat 2001).

- **Imagination**: some people find that talking is more difficult than other means of communication, such as drawing, singing, dancing, showing, etc., so you need to provide many possibilities for creative expression of memories.

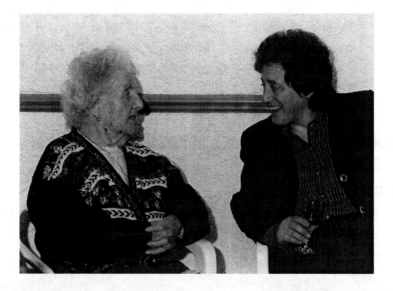

Figure 3.2: Gertie enjoys singing remembered songs with Pam, even though she now finds talking difficult

When working with a group, there are additional requirements:

- **A degree of self-confidence**: you must be willing to take the lead in some activities, so people in the group understand what you are suggesting, to steer and refocus the conversation where necessary and to take some risks.

- **A democratic approach**: everyone's contributions must be valued and people with dementia must be given plenty of opportunity and extra time to contribute.

- **Group work skills**: there are always links and connections between what different group members say, however different their backgrounds may be. Good facilitation involves pointing up these links for the group and creating a sense of shared experience and common ground.

- **Caring**: there is a responsibility to take care of the emotional needs of group members. If someone is distressed, time should be made for them to talk (if necessary after the session) and extra help made available if required.

- **Practicality**: the physical needs of the group must be considered, so that everyone can hear and see everyone else in the session. Facilitators need to be alert to needs of individuals and ensure that they can participate, so, for example, people who are hard of hearing should be seated near or opposite the group leader and the group leader should speak clearly.

TRIGGERING MEMORIES, ESPECIALLY THROUGH SENSORY STIMULI

Objects

An object will bring back memories because of the way it looks and feels, its weight and texture. Finding the right objects for each person takes time and

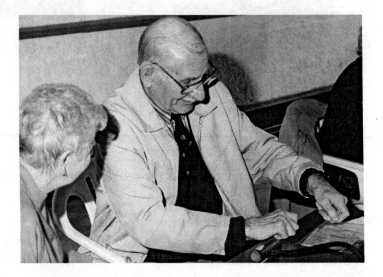

Figure 3.3: Jim demonstrates the docker's technique of lifting heavy goods with a docker's hook

can involve visits to markets, museums and boot sales. For example old work tools or garden equipment can be powerful reminders of earlier days and people will often enjoy handling them again and showing how they used them, even if speech or powers of description are limited. Finding appropriate items is a task the family might help with if they are still involved and willing to bring things along from home.

Using work tools as a stimulus

Jim worked in the docks all his life and was very knowledgeable about cargos and how to move impossibly heavy bags from one place to another. Given a docker's hook (the tool used to lift hundredweight bags of sugar onto the quay) he could speak eloquently about the task, supporting his description with the physical actions so well remembered by his body. Though he had difficulty remembering many things, especially those relating to the very recent past, these memories were crystallised through years of experience and served him well to communicate with others in the present.

Photos

Photographs can also be enlarged and used to trigger memories. This enlargement reveals details not normally visible and it is often these details which are needed to strike a chord, for example, a wallpaper pattern, a favourite dress, a pair of shoes or a swimming costume. The best results have

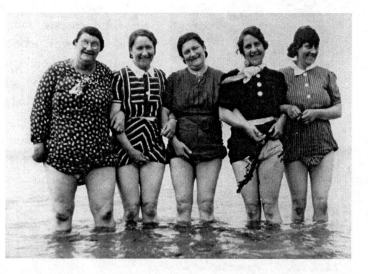

Figure 3.4: Gertie recognised all her sisters when this seaside photo from long ago was enlarged for her

been produced by taking copyshots of originals with a digital camera and enlarging them. However, up-to-date photocopiers can often produce a good result.

Enlarging a photo

Edith's daughter Pat went through the family photos and found a tiny snap of her mother and a pet dog when she was a little girl. She brought the photo in so it could be enlarged. The following week, Pat showed the enlarged photo to Edith, saying 'Look at this Mum. Is that little girl you? I wonder where it was taken?' Edith looked at the photo for quite a time before pointing at the floor tiles clearly visible in the enlarged photo, saying 'That's my Grandma's house, it must be, I know the pattern on her floor.' Edith kept having another look at the photo and remembering more. She noticed the buttons on her shoes, and remembered how hard they were to do up. 'And that's me with the dog.' Pat wrote a letter to the project leader after this session, including the following: 'Have put as much information as we have gleaned on the back of the photograph. The real gem was recalling the name of the dog. The dog was called Radio after the cat's whisker radio which my grandfather proudly bought and which I believe my mother has drawn in one of her "sketches from childhood" a few weeks back.'

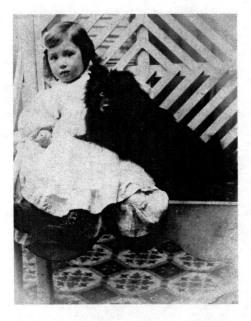

Photographs which are relevant to a person's life story are particularly productive, such as the street he or she grew up in, his or her places of work, the local cinema, family occasions. Wedding photos, school photos and photos of works outings show people from past times who may be well remembered. Again, relatives can be helpful with resources and ideas, and local libraries can often provide large black and white photos of local firms and recorded events.

Figure 3.5: Edith, aged 91, recognises her very young self and remembers the dog and the floor tiles when the photo is enlarged

---

Where I used to work

When Tom's key worker Sue asked him about his life, he told her that he was apprenticed at Dean's foundry when he was 14 and worked there for 30 years. Sue had never heard of Dean's but asked around, and found out that the foundry had closed years ago, and the building had been demolished. She went to the library, and the librarian helped her find some local history books. In one of them there was a photo of Dean's in 1935, the year after Tom started there. She copied the photo and showed it to Tom who recognised it at once, and told her a lot more about working at Dean's. She found a frame for it and gave it to Tom who enjoyed showing it to visitors and asking them if they remembered Dean's Foundry.

Smells

Smells, both pleasant and unpleasant, can be a very effective means of stimulating memories. Flowers, vegetables and herbs can evoke memories of early life experience and of hobbies and enthusiasms of later life.

Lavender's blue

An elderly man living in sheltered housing in Hackney smelled lavender and came forth with a childhood memory of living in France with his grandma who always had lavender in her linen cupboard. He described the layers of white starched sheets in the tall wooden wardrobe which smelt wonderful, and then went on to explain that actually she was quite cruel and his French childhood had been traumatic. He attended an RYCT project with his son who came to the housing complex to take part. The son talked about not normally having very much communication with his father, and said that the structured programme enabled them to move beyond their usual pattern of communication.

Strong smells associated with childhood such as camphorated oil, carbolic soap or Mansion polish can trigger memories of family life and routines and rituals. Well-known perfumes such as 4711 or Evening in Paris (or maybe Brylcream for men) can be powerful reminders of youthful flirtations and courting days.

Strong smells…and not always pleasant ones!

A woman visiting the Reminiscence Centre in London with a group from her care home was exploring a big chest of drawers, such as might be found in an old 'oil shop' or general store with small objects in every drawer. She happened upon a drawer with mothballs in it and the strong smell of naphtha transported her back to childhood days and her mother's wardrobe where she used to like to play sometimes. This woman rarely spoke, but she said 'Mothballs!' and was clearly pleased to be able to voice her memory.

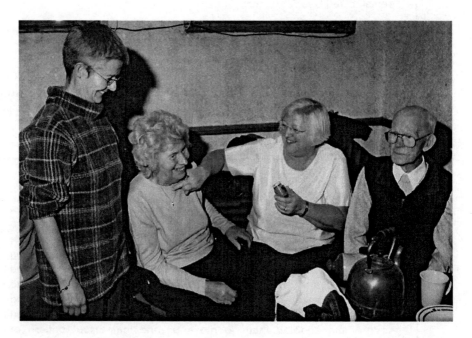

Figure 3.6: Prompting memories of winter remedies by stimulating the sense of smell

Tastes

Simple things like old-fashioned sweets with wrappings can evoke memories, including where the local sweetshop was, what you could get in the war years and what people spent their pocket money on. Old recipes, perhaps associated with austerity years or with special occasions in the year, can be located in cookery books and even tried out for taste. Again, families can be helpful here. Perhaps they remember the person's favourite foods and can write down remembered meals to go in a personal recipe booklet. Having an old-fashioned tea with scones and china cups can give a sense of occasion, and if there is a family who, for example, remember Gran's famous chocolate cake, they can make one to her recipe to bring in, and it will certainly add something special to the event.

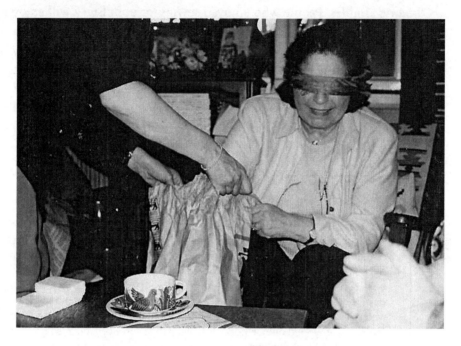

Figure 3.7: Stimulating the senses with a 'touchy-feely' bag in the Brussels RYCT group

Textures and touch

Women often gain satisfaction from handling fabrics which they might have sewn or worn, especially fabrics which are less common today. Saying the names of the fabrics and exploring old dress patterns can bring back many memories.

The feel of silk

When a silk evening dress from the 1930s was put into Zita's lap, her eyes lit up as she felt the fabric. She said: 'I had one like this. It was a short one. Shell-pink. It was rather revealing. I used to like it – my mother used to say "you can't wear that!"' Zita went on to recall further details about wearing her dress – it was sleeveless and looked best if you didn't wear anything with it, and she wore shoes with ankle straps and heels, not high heels, just little ones. She wore it to go dancing, which she loved.

People often remember where they bought clothes in the past or where they bought the fabric to make them themselves. It is often worth making up a sewing box with cotton reels, darning wool, thimbles, needles, patches and fabric samples. People who enjoyed sewing or upholstery will enjoy rummaging in the box and sorting through the items. Fur coats and satin or velvet dresses are particularly pleasurable to handle, and it is not always necessary to ask people to voice the thoughts such things might trigger. They may just enjoy holding the dress up against themselves and doing a twirl, or putting a fur stole over their shoulders and feeling glamorous, especially if it evokes 'the feel' of the past. Wedding clothes especially can be very evocative.

Wedding day clothes

In a session on weddings, two ladies brought in items they had worn on their wedding days. One was a veil in a very soft material, lovely to feel. She put it on her head, without covering her face, to tell us her wedding memory. The other lady allowed her dress to be passed around the group and each person held it up against them while they described what they wore on their wedding day. This sometimes included suits or costumes worn at wartime weddings when suitable bridal dresses were in short supply. It seemed that holding up the real dress reminded people not only of what they had worn, but also how they had felt about it at the time.

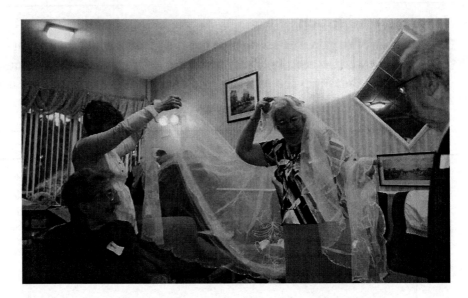

Figure 3.8: Eva remembers her own wedding day, and the veil which she has kept

Sounds

Tapes or CDs of sounds such as bird song, brass bands, church bells, or even sea and rain, are available from libraries. We can experiment to find out which sounds are evocative for particular people. Railway enthusiasts usually love train noises, bird watchers might like tapes of bird song to identify calls and interpret particular sounds. Short extracts from recordings like these can be useful as a stimulus for group or one-to-one discussion.

It is also fun to make a sound collage with a group of people related to a theme. Provided this is treated lightly and explained as a quirky way to stimulate mind pictures of past events to share, people will often participate with pleasure.

Sound collages

A whole group of older women from China made sound collages about their childhoods in three different locations: by the sea with all its steamers, hooters, birds and waves; in the city with the traffic noises, trains, shouting and market traders and in the country, with bird song, crops swaying and 'whispering' in the wind, animals calling and even the chomping of mulberry leaves by silkworms on a silk farm! The way this worked was that each person said something about the place where they grew up and the rest of the group responded by guessing if this or that sound would be heard there. The person said yes or no, and gradually everyone had an appropriate sound they could add in. The session leader conducted the sound collage, with people adding their sound when the leader called them in, with loud and soft versions of each sound.

This proved a powerful trigger to further memories, even with one lady, Choi Wah Liu, whose powers of recall were very limited. Stimulated by sounds made by the group of the mulberry leaves being eaten by the silk worms and the fish coming to the surface in the large pond on the farm, she then recalled her father carrying her on his shoulders when she was very young and the sound of his feet on the ground as he walked, which of course the group added into the sound collage. This lady went on to make a beautiful memory box about her life with help from an artist and working through an interpreter.

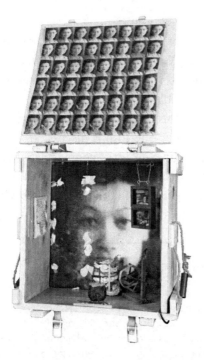

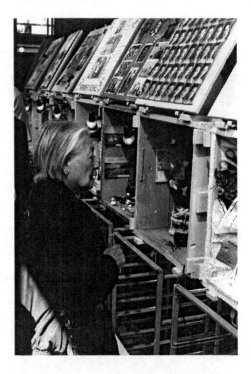

Figure 3.9a: Choi Wah Liu's memory box based on memories of the Chinese silk farm where she grew up

Figure 3.9b: Choi Wah Liu looks into her memory box on display and it helps her remember her own story all over again

Music

Music and songs from earlier times in life are a powerful stimulus, and often trigger associated memories of social occasions, significant days and relationships (Aldridge 2000; Greenyer 2003). Singing familiar songs together can help build a sense of group identity and belonging. People with dementia will often remember the words of songs and enjoy singing even when speech has become problematical. A group can try to remember all the words of a song, by pooling the bits they remember and writing them down, then singing them again together. Humming along, whistling the tune or tapping out the rhythm are all valid ways of contributing and enjoying the music together.

It is always worth trying to find out about what a particular person enjoys, so that you do not assume too much. Often there are surprises, such as finding someone has been a lifelong opera enthusiast or a lover of contemporary pop music. Some people have belonged to choirs and orchestras and have retained their capacity to read notes, even when the reading of text is difficult.

'Didn't we sing well?'

Edith had always enjoyed singing in a choir. On her 90th birthday she held a harmony line with the group leader and her daughter, to everyone's surprise and delight. Her daughter wrote: 'What a wonderful afternoon we had yesterday, meeting up again with the Remembering Yesterday, Caring Today group and celebrating Edith's 90th birthday. Thank you all so much... And didn't we sing well!?'

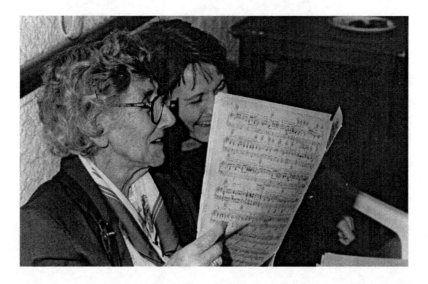

Figure 3.10: Edith remembers how to read music and shares her skill with Hannah, a volunteer

Making a Desert Island Discs-style compilation tape or CD of a person's favourite songs is quite an undertaking, but the response is likely to be very positive. Such a tape can then be a jumping-off point for further reminiscence, and these associated memories too can be recorded against a time when they are no longer so easily recalled (at which time they will make pleasurable and recognisable listening).

Dancing

The body has its memory for steps, movements and rhythms (Violets-Gibson 2004). Prompted by appropriate music, live or recorded, people with dementia can often dance more competently than their carers supposed possible (Coaten 2001). Where this is no longer possible, people can find great pleasure in watching others dance, remembering past pleasures of their own.

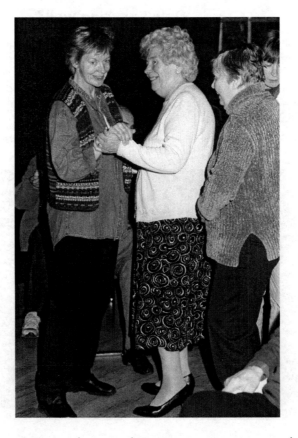

Figure 3.11: Margaret enjoys dancing with Anny Evason, an RYCT group leader

Shall we dance?

Margaret, a lady with quite advanced dementia who rarely uttered a word in conversation in our group, but communicated with body language and facial expressions, danced with a reminiscence worker to a slow wartime love song, smiling and singing the words of the song as they danced – while clearly enjoying her own memories.

And Amy, who had not danced with her husband Reg for ten years, joined in the session on dancing memories with great happiness. She held tight to Reg as they danced, she nodded when the dance hall where they met was named, and at the end of the dance they kissed, to great applause from the rest of the group.

Enactment as a reminiscence trigger

Because enactment stimulates so many senses simultaneously, it is particularly effective with people with dementia (Batson 1998; Schweitzer 2007). When we invite people to revisit a memory as though it is happening in the present, we are inviting spontaneous responses to verbal, kinaesthetic (movement), oral, and often musical and textural prompts as well. We are not in 'quiz' mode, asking questions which have danger of failure attached to them, where only a few people can do well and which rely heavily on a verbal response. We are setting up an 'as if' situation for the person or group to respond to in ways which feel appropriate to them and which are not right or wrong. By recreating familiar past situations in the present, we are enabling people to call on their personal lived experience and to participate as equals in bringing these situations alive.

Virtual holiday-making

In a session on holidays, we drew a chalk map on the floor and scattered the chairs around the perimeter. We indicated that different parts of the room represented holiday destinations and invited people to sit in an area of which they had fond memories. In this way, people who had holidayed in the Lake District, the Isle of Man, the Kent coast, or even the Caribbean had a place to go and sit, often with people who shared good memories of those places. They were then asked to group themselves into 'still photos' of remembered scenes and show them to the whole group. This prompted much recognition and recall of familiar situations and a lot of laughter and good humour. Some of these photos were then 'brought to life' in the groups, with help from workers and volunteers. When Margaret did not feel able to play herself, Viv, a worker, took her part, asking her for ideas about how it was, and checking back with her on everything she did, so it could feel right to Margaret as the originator. Each small group shared their, often hilarious, scenes with the whole group, and by the end of the afternoon many people felt they had been on holiday!

Some facilitators have shied away from using enactment as they have felt they lacked the necessary charisma to 'pull it off', but when they have taken the risk, they have found it to be a particularly effective way of engaging the people with dementia, and their own confidence in the method has rapidly increased.

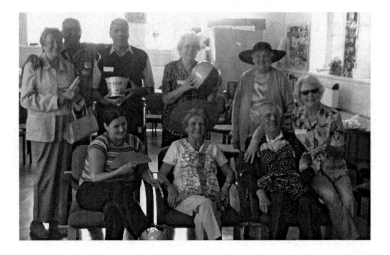

Figure 3.12: Group photo of a virtual trip to the seaside with the Bradford RYCT group

Taking the plunge

I wasn't confident about enactments – I didn't think I could act and so didn't feel easy about asking anyone else to do it (imagining they would feel the same).

This changed after I went on a day's training and was forced(!) to have a go. We'd been asked to share memories about Sundays and mine was about being in church with my sisters. We sat very near Miss Brown, the organist, who perched on a stool and played the hymns on a small organ – every week the combination of her seriousness and the strange squeakings and groanings which accompanied her playing sent us into uncontrollable giggles. Enacting it brought the memory back in a very real way with the added pleasure of doing it with others – it made me feel very good that they chose my story to play out and it showed me that it's not really about acting so much as being able to relax with other people and have fun – the fact that it's your memory makes that (and you) feel quite special.

Later when I was facilitating a group of carers who were sharing memories of their schooldays, I felt much more confident about encouraging them to enact their memories. I remember one carer in particular who told us a story about bringing in his grandad's false teeth to school and using them to disrupt a class. With a little encouragement, he 'let go' and really played to the house (much better than I could!). There was a lot of laughter and looking back it was probably the best moment in the project.

Being prepared to try enactments feels risky but is in fact very unlikely to fail. Making mistakes doesn't matter and the experience makes the whole group feel good. It's both about being able to be silly with other people, and the more serious element of valuing someone's memory and how that makes that person feel.

(Sarah Hodgson, group leader)

Words and sayings

In the normal course of conversation between the person with dementia and the carer, spontaneous memories often emerge. Writing these down and typing them out in large print to put up on the walls (with the person's permission of course) can help that person to feel good about what he or she has remembered and can give others ideas for conversation.

Recorded messages from the family reminding their relative of enjoyable past times together can be fun to make and pleasing for the relative to listen to as often as he or she likes. The messages can be chatty in style, like a typical telephone conversation, with an affectionate message and some personal reflections and graphic reminders. This approach was originally based on the idea that people with dementia who are missing their families might find it reassuring to hear the voice of someone who matters to them. It is known as 'simulated presence therapy', and studies have shown that for some people it works very well. Interestingly, it has been found that people often respond to the recording as if it were a real telephone conversation, so it is important that it is made with pauses which allow time for the person listening to respond (Peak and Cheston 2002).

Example of a taped message

'Hello Mum, it's Maggie. I hope you are well today. (Pause) I've just been remembering the holiday we had in Wales when I was little. Do you remember that? (Pause) We went to Rhyl and stayed at The Waves Guest House in Sea Road. (Pause) We had those little rooms in the attic, you loved the blue walls and white woodwork, do you remember? (Pause) We could watch the pigeons on the roof-tops from the attic windows. They were so funny, we used to laugh at them strutting about puffing their chests out. (Pause) We were on the beach every day, rain or shine. (Pause) I've just found a photo of us sitting on the beach in our cardies, all wrapped up. You had a towel over your legs like a blanket. (Pause) I wonder if you remember the old windbreak with blue and orange stripes? We had that for years? (Pause) We had such lovely times at Rhyl.'

Old proverbs and well-worn phrases often trigger memories of elderly relatives or parents who used them a lot. It is fun to make a list and say them together.

Proverbs

People will sometimes remember quite a lot of sayings their parents and grandparents used to use. In a big group, one such memory will trigger another, and each will have memories attached relating to the speaker and the situation. For example, one person remembering her grandmother saying 'Waste not, want not' led to her recalling some of the extraordinary things her grandmother refused to throw away and the resulting chaos in her house. Another remembered her mother saying 'A bird in the hand is worth two in the bush,' and using this proverb to try to get her daughter to settle for a boyfriend who was certainly not the husband of her dreams!

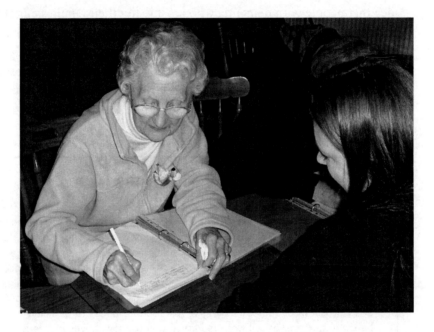

Figure 3.13: Writing down a memory recaptured with support from a volunteer

Writing

Some people still enjoy writing, and others appreciate having someone write for them. Writing a note to a friend remembered in a reminiscence exercise can be a way of expressing feelings of fondness, even if the letter does not get sent as there is no longer contact in reality. Offering to write down a message or memory for someone with dementia who has just remembered a friend or relative with pleasure (or indeed with anger or sadness) can be an equally satisfying way of expressing important feelings in the present.

Poetry

Many people who learned whole poems by heart when they were at school still remember them and enjoy reciting them together. Others enjoy listening to familiar poems as recited or read by others, and will join in where they can. What one person forgets, another remembers, so a small group can sometimes find all the lines of a well-known poem such as Wordsworth's 'Daffodils' or John Masefield's 'Sea Fever', write them down and then say them together.

Some carers and people with dementia have found writing poetry to be an important means of expressing the changes they are experiencing. Joan Sharp, a family carer, wrote the following poem about coming to terms with her husband's dementia. When her poem was read out to the group, it helped others to share their own inner struggles. This is what she wrote:

> Remembering yesterday, caring today
> That says it all in a new kind of way.
> For remembering has given so much to me,
> Reassurance, a direction, greater sensibility.
> I now have another challenge in my life,
> Not only being a loving, caring wife.
> I never thought I could feel this way,
> I'm thinking of things I just have to say.
> Putting it in verse, I would never have dreamt
> So thanks to the project,
> Every word I say is meant.
>
> My husband's needs must come first now
> For in sickness and in health I took a vow.
> I will come to terms with this illness,
> Even though I still don't know how.
>
> The project has taught me so many things,
> To have patience and think of others' feelings.
> Get down to their level when sitting in a chair,
> Hold hands, say your name, to let them know who's there.
> Speak softly and slowly, never ever shout,
> Don't reprimand: they don't know what they're about.

Our tête-à-têtes are now in the past,
But you do give me signs that I understand,
The special look, with that cheeky smile,
And a warm squeeze of the hand.

The love we have together,
Will be with us till we part,
Till my strength gives up on me,
I'll be there, sweetheart.

Warriors and Battlers

written by John Barclay on 18th October 2005

We are the broken and damaged
but with the help of the great fraternity,
fraternity of the warriors of the blue elephant
and the battlers from Llandygai,
we may not fly like eagles but we will keep our dignity.
When the great Amen has sounded
we will have kept our dignity.
When the knell has sounded
we will have kept our dignity.[1]

This was written by John during the course of the project. After he had been diagnosed with a form of dementia, he decided that he would not be able to write poetry any more. He had lost a lifelong hobby and much of the confidence he had previously had. After much encouragement he produced this poem as a gift to our Dementia Services Development Centre and for me to use in my teaching. He has since written more poems and has become an active member of the North Wales Forum for people with dementia.

(Joan Woods, Bangor RYCT group leader)

[1]   'Blue elephant' was the name of the bus that took the people to the weekly sessions. Llandygai is the name of the place where they met.

Selective use of radio and television

Using the *Radio Times* or other listings to locate programmes of music and memories connected with the interests of the person can give listening to radio and watching television considerably more meaning and purpose.

Videos, CDs or DVDs are just as useful for this sort of activity, with the added advantage that they can be stopped and replayed at particularly

---

Television can be interesting!

A carer who was depressed by the sight of her husband sitting blankly in front of the television decided to try another approach. She talked him through the day's offerings, especially highlighting programmes relating to military matters and famous battles, and only turned the television on for those programmes. She sat with him to watch and turned the set off afterwards to talk a little about what they had watched together.

---

interesting moments. People who have been musicians may enjoy clips of themselves playing, or others playing their favourite pieces.

Computer programs

There are some computer programs designed to aid reminiscence. For example, CIRCA is an interactive program using reminiscence to stimulate conversation with family or paid carers. It has been designed specially for people with dementia and it can successfully engage their attention and interest. Experience with CIRCA shows that many people with dementia can learn to interact with the system using a touch screen (Alm *et al.* 2007). Acting Up: Multimedia For a Change also provides multimedia training and support for people with communication difficulties. See www.actingup.org.uk.

Visits

It is worth making the effort to take people out to visit the places where they went to school or danced or worked, or worshipped and married, if such places are still standing. Such visits in the present also offer a storehouse of new memories to talk about in the future.

Going back to 'the big house'

A lady who was taken to visit 'the big house' where she worked in service from the age of 13, found she could remember a great deal about the people and the place in 'her time'. In this instance, the house was still in the same family's ownership and a care worker was able to organise the visit. The family encouraged the old lady to go round the house, finding all the familiar bits, and everyone got something out of the experience.

Visits to museums of everyday life in earlier decades can stir many memories and some museums are particularly welcoming to groups of older people. They may even make available items from their 'handling collections' to stimulate a discussion. But even if it is just a matter of looking together at carefully arranged displays of objects arranged thematically, such an outing can be very enjoyable, an effective stimulus and something to look back on with pleasure as a group or as a family.

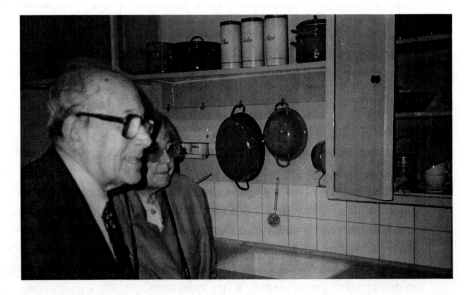

Figure 3.14: Members of the RYCT group in Amsterdam enjoy a visit to their local museum of everyday life

Inter-generational work

Inter-generational work makes use of the natural inclination for older people to pass on their experience to the young, and the delight that many older people have in contact with babies and young children. People with dementia can participate successfully in inter-generational work and benefit from contact with babies and children (Woodhead 2004). Many homes have visits from school groups who perform songs or nativity plays at Christmas, and there is scope to make this more of a two-way process by encouraging the audience to give something back to the children, as organisations like Magic Me (www.magicme.co.uk) and Age Exchange (www.age-exchange.org.uk) have shown.

Contact with babies and young children can be an uplifting experience for some people with dementia, and trigger many memories. Although dolls make a convenient substitute, the sound, smell and feel of a real baby stimulates the senses in a way that a doll does not. When old people react appropriately and spontaneously to young people, they remind themselves and those around them, that they too were once carers, and competent ones at that.

It is worth remembering that not-so-young grandchildren and other younger members of the family can be valuable volunteers if reminiscence products are being made, and many have invaluable computer skills to create interesting collages and interactive visual reminiscence prompts.

BACKGROUND RESEARCH FOR SUCCESSFUL REMINISCENCE WORK

Reminiscence workers need to have and show a real interest in the times their people have lived through and the places they have come from. Hearing people's stories can whet our appetites to know more, and the more we follow this interest through the more effective we can be as questioners, listeners and prompters.

History

Care workers who have increased their knowledge of recent social and cultural history have found this to be a valuable key to engaging in talking about a person's past life experience. The people who now have dementia have lived through the major events of the twentieth century, the Depression, World War II, the austerity period, and the greater freedom of the 1960s. Knowing something about the historical context, through books, films and documentaries, can enable carers to ask more relevant questions, prompt more effectively and understand the answers better.

Learning all about it

Dorothy kept talking about her time in the Land Army. Kevin, born in 1981, had no idea what this was, and Dorothy was not able to explain it clearly, but told him it was during the war. He was not even sure which war she meant. His head of home lent him a video of *The Land Girls* which he enjoyed watching. This gave him important background information and insight into how it might have felt to be a young London girl suddenly transported to the different world of the Shropshire countryside. Dorothy was away from her family for the first time and dealing with unfamiliar animals, large and small, and learning to use agricultural tools and machines.

When caring for someone from another culture, we are even more likely to be ignorant about his or her country and its history. A small amount of time spent on the Internet, or looking at other sources to find out something about the way of life and important events in that country, can make a big difference to our understanding of the person's background. It is very comforting for people growing old in a strange country to feel that they are speaking to someone with some inkling of their past life and circumstances.

Finding out about a different history

Mai Lee fled Vietnam on a small boat bound for Hong Kong with only a few family photos and a blanket. Now in her 80s, she was attending a London day centre for people with dementia. Irene, the activities worker, felt that she needed to understand more about Mai's situation at that time, so she searched the web under 'Vietnam' and 'Boat People' and found a wealth of information, historical detail and personal stories. This helped her to understand what Mai had had to deal with and to ask her more appropriate questions. It also helped her to understand Mai's current fears and feelings.

Language

The day-to-day language we use is of its time and we need to be sensitive to this when engaging with much older people. There will be words and phrases they use which mean nothing to us, and vice-versa, and we need to be aware of the potential gulf here.

Oops... I got it wrong

Jenny was involved in a reminiscence session on daily life in the 1920s and 1930s, when people in the group were children. Nell mentioned going every week to the pawn shop for her mother. Jenny was not at all sure how to respond to this, as she thought Nell was referring to a porn shop. She wondered why on earth the mother sent her child along, but did not like to ask. Only in discussion after the session was it explained to her by another worker that this was a service used a lot by poorer families who needed cash in a hurry. They left items of some value, a suit, a watch, a wedding ring, and received money on loan in exchange. They could then retrieve these items at a later date when they repaid the money with interest, after payday or a Christmas bonus payout. Everyone laughed about the misunderstanding but it was a useful lesson about making sure you are speaking the same language.

It is worthwhile asking people to explain something we have not understood as, even if they are not able to do this, it does show a willingness to listen and understand. Also, when engaging someone in conversation, perhaps on a new topic concerned with the past, it is worth expressing things more than once, choosing different words to elucidate, as this gives people more than one chance to get our drift.

WORKING ACROSS CULTURES

We need to recognise the importance of cultural background to the different people we are working with, and take the trouble to find out something about it. For example, in all cultures the year is marked by seasons and significant, often religious, festivals. In each culture these have actions, phrases and songs connected to them which an old person with dementia can often perform confidently. The performance of the actions and the reciting of prayers, greetings and praises may activate intact personal memories and associations, which a worker can draw out in conversation with the person. The more familiar the worker can become with the calendar events and the associated rituals which have shaped the lives of the people he or she is working with, the more appropriate prompts can be produced, the more responses can be understood, and the more successful and rewarding the reminiscence work is likely to be.

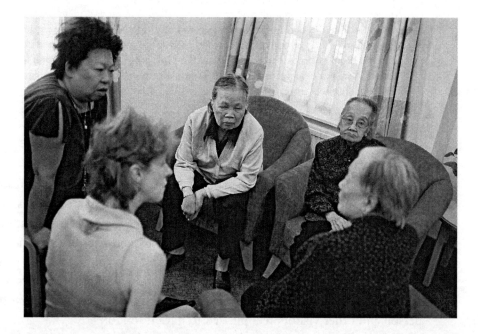

Figure 3.15: Chinese elders in London remembering in a group and preparing to make a scene from their memories with help from Sharon Morgan, RYCT group leader

When working in a multicultural group, it is important to enable people to mark the festivals that are important to them. Many of these will be equivalent to our own festivals and happen at similar times of year, for example spring ceremonials at Easter, harvest-related autumn festivals, and festivals of light in the winter. We can invite people to share their customs with us. Celebrating difference in this way often has the effect of making everyone in a group feel special and interesting, as though the whole world is in the room together and that they as individuals and as a group have a special value. The more these celebrations of seasons and life passage rituals can be performed and brought to life, the more vivid people's memories will be and the more effective these life course and seasonal milestones will be as memory triggers benefiting the whole group (Schweitzer 2004).

Celebrating difference

When it came to the session on weddings, Noriko, a Japanese post-graduate student, prepared a presentation for the group to show what a wedding was like in her country. She wore a special kimono and explained the rituals of the courting and marriage ceremonies, and sang a special wedding song. Everyone in the group was enchanted, listening avidly and thanking her. This opened the door for many wedding stories from the different cultures present in the group. Maria, originally from Spain, led us all in a village wedding dance, teaching us the tune and some of the steps. We moved on to perform essential elements of a Jewish wedding ceremony together, with an improvised Chuppa (wedding canopy), represented by a large towel held up on sticks! and the ritual of breaking a glass under the bridegroom's heel. Everyone felt included in performing one another's rituals and enriched by the cultural variety within the group.

MAKING REMINISCENCE PRODUCTS

Making reminiscence products can be very rewarding, but we must be realistic about the amount of time it can take. Life story books, memory boxes, collages and displays are examples of different ways to record reminiscence work. For example making a collage of photos and captions over a few weeks with help from family members can result in an attractive wall panel which will also serve as a stimulus for conversation with other visitors. It is important to do this with some care and make it look attractive so that the person and other visitors feel pleased to have it to look at.

Life story products can also be a very important resource, particularly at a time of change, for example when someone goes into long-term care or into

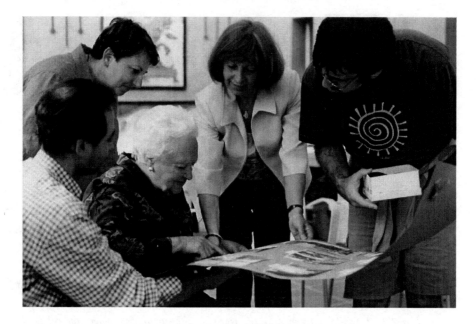

Figure 3.16: A personal photomontage in the Barcelona RYCT project

Personal photomontages

Sandy Foster in Australia used collage photo-boards to stimulate much conversation and exchange and also to help other staff to learn more about the real enthusiasms (past and present) of their residents. Photos with captions were attractively arranged on a coloured background and put on the person's wall to stimulate dialogue and to remind all visitors that the person they were visiting had had a full and interesting life. One man's panel was all about horses, about which he was extremely knowledgeable. He liked having the pictures and stories in his room and his visitors found the photo-board to be a useful starting point for conversation.

hospital. At times like this a life story book, memory box or collage can provide a link between past and present, giving new care workers an insight into the person they are caring for. These products are usually valued by family members both during the person's lifetime and after he or she has died. There have even been occasions when a person's memory box has been a centre-piece at their funeral service, where friends and family have found it helpful to have reminders of the person and a special personal life portrait to discuss together.

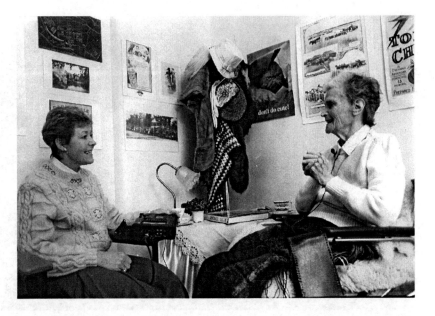

Figure 3.17: Sandy Foster in Australia working with stimulating images and enlarged photos, recording a resident's memories

Making and showing a memory box

Noel made a memory box about his life, helped by an artist. Over a series of one-to-one sessions with the artist, in which Noel's wife played a supporting role, Noel told stories, drew his memories and found photos and small objects relating to different aspects of his life in the Caribbean and in London. Together with the artist he assembled these drawings, photos and objects into a 3-D collage featuring his Caribbean background and his love of campervan holidays with his wife in England, with their sense of freedom and the open road. It also featured his marriage to his London-born wife.

On their wedding anniversary which coincided with a group meeting, the box was brought to the session and provided a lively half hour of questions, answers and story-telling which was pleasurable for all and extremely gratifying for Noel and his wife. He rose to the occasion splendidly and enabled everyone present to sense what was important to him and what was special about him. So what began as a one-to-one reminiscence process became a product, the memory box, which could then be shared with a wider group. As time has gone on, Noel has found drawing and talking more difficult, but he can still remember many things about his life with the evidence from his memory box in front of him.

Deciding whether your work is about the process (valuing the moment) or product (working towards an addition to the records, a life story book, display, collage, etc.) or a combination of both is an issue for any kind of reminiscence work, planned or unplanned, group or individual. Sometimes, what begins as a plan to hold a couple of trial sessions then becomes a more ambitious joint undertaking with an unexpected end-product.

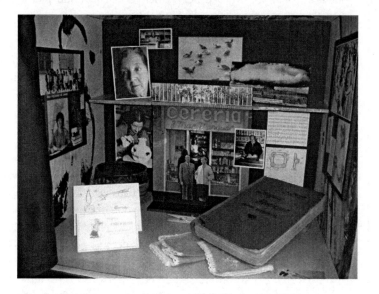

Figure 3.18: A memory box created in Barcelona from one family's memories

LEARNING FROM EXPERIENCE AND EVALUATION

We need to observe what happens during reminiscence work, and afterwards think about how things went for the people we are working with and evaluate the activities we used (Johns 2000). It is not always easy to take in everything that happens as we go along, and it can be useful to have someone taking the role of observer from time to time.

It is a good idea to think about the aims of each reminiscence session. Having aims is helpful when evaluating the work. General aims for reminiscence work are:

- to do something that engages people with dementia

- to foster communication and conversation

- to create a lively atmosphere

- to show that people, and their stories, are valued.

Having an observer

BACKGROUND

A group activity in the lounge of Greenhill House (a unit for people with dementia) took place after mid-morning coffee on a morning when everything had gone smoothly, residents were up and dressed and two staff realised that there was time for a group activity before lunch. A gap year student on a volunteer programme was asked to act as observer.

ACTIVITY

Reminiscence using a box of objects associated with washing and mending – including carbolic soap, washboard, penny blue, darning mushroom, thimble, pin-cushion and darning wool.

OBSERVER'S NOTES

It's really good that there was time for an activity this morning. Edith and Joan's faces lit up when it was suggested. Getting people into a circle for the activity meant getting people to move and some of them weren't very keen on this. We didn't push it, but the resulting problem was that some of them couldn't see and hear what was going on very well.

Everyone was given an object from the box to look at. Some people were much more interested in their objects than others. It reminded me of a classroom quiz when each person was asked to say if they remembered what their object was. Sophie had the pin-cushion, and made everyone laugh pretending it was a hedgehog. She told us all about doing this with her Nan when she was little. Bill and Nettie chipped in with memories about their grandparents, and there was a lively chat. But not everyone was engaged in this.

Sophie had a lovely time. She had lots of memories and listened to what other people were saying with interest.

Bill, Nettie, Edith and Joan also seemed to enjoy the activity. They were all able to say something about the objects they were given. Bill made a joke about his, and then told us about working extra shifts when saving up for a twin-tub for his wife. Amazing to hear him say so much! (Bill is only 68, so some of these objects were a bit old fashioned for him?) Nettie lost interest when the people who were talking were too far away and she couldn't hear what they were saying. Edith remembered using darning mushrooms at school, and then told us about the schoolroom. She looked a bit crestfallen when she was reminded that we weren't supposed to be talking about school.

Mary was holding the bar of carbolic soap. When she was asked to say what it was, she was tongue-tied. She did eventually say something, but everyone was listening to Bill by that time. She didn't look very happy.

Beryl sat there stroking the sampler she had been given, looking very sad. I thought she might cry at any minute. She was never asked to say anything because the activity had to end suddenly when the staff were called away. (But I stopped being the observer at that point and was able to talk to her. She did cry, telling me about her mother and older sister dying within a month of each other when she was 12, but she said she liked to talk about them even though it made her cry.)

During a quiet moment towards the end of the shift, the staff asked the volunteer what she had observed. She started with positive points, then mentioned what she had noticed about Mary and Beryl. Together they thought about different ways of organising the activity to make it work better.

We can think about specific aims for particular people, and these do not have to be ambitious. For example, we might simply aim to elicit a response from a person who is very withdrawn, or to get a smile from someone (Heathcote 2007). In Chapter 5 we offer some specific advice on evaluating RYCT projects.

Chapter 4

Remembering Yesterday, Caring Today

A Programme and an Approach

THE RYCT APPROACH

Remembering Yesterday, Caring Today is both a specific programme and an approach to reminiscence that can be used more widely. The RYCT approach combines good practice in reminiscence with the person-centred approach to dementia care. Its starting point is creative arts-based reminiscence work,

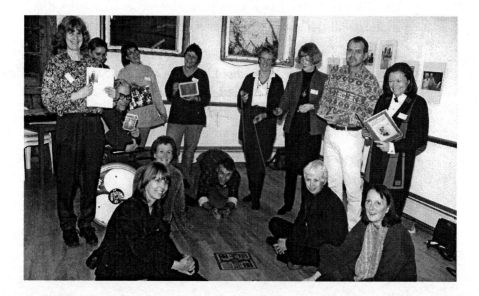

Figure 4.1: Partners piloting the original RYCT project undergo experiential training in London exploring their own memories of childhood in response to reminiscence triggers

with an emphasis on multi-sensory stimulation and non-verbal channels of communication. Woven into this is the recognition that we can add value to reminiscence activities by creating opportunities for the different types of positive interaction described by Kitwood (1997) as positive person work.

Creative reminiscence gives considerable scope for positive interactions involving, for example, recognition, collaboration, sensory stimulation, validation, celebration and playfulness. Perrin and May's (2000) discussion of the 'playful practitioner' and the value of humour, spontaneity and joy for people with dementia is a reminder of the difference between worthy but unimaginative reminiscence and the approach we are describing here.

The RYCT programme has also been run successfully in groups where family carers have not attended, and we have included a section on adapting the sessions for what we have called 'reminiscence alone' groups. Many of the small group activities developed for each reminiscence theme have also been successfully used or adapted in one-to-one situations both at home and in care homes.

Key features of the RYCT approach

- Working in ways that enable people with dementia to participate fully in reminiscence work, and to feel valued and fully included.

- Using a structured approach to reminiscence and activities that stimulate all the senses to trigger memories.

- Making use of the creative arts – music, sound, visual arts, photography, dance, movement, writing and drama – to give added value to stories told, to facilitate full use of non-verbal expression, to provide outlets for creativity and humour and to create a 'doing' atmosphere.

- Creating opportunities for interactions and activities that enhance the well-being of participants with dementia.

- Sharing common experience and celebrating differences.

- Having a supportive attitude to family carers and their relationships with those they are caring for, whether or not family carers are actively involved.

- When working in groups, giving participants the opportunity to get to know one another by working together, providing a sense of belonging and friendship at a time when this is particularly necessary.

The handout 'Guidelines for RYCT project leaders and volunteers' (see Appendix) lists essential ways of working which help the project teams following the RYCT programme to put the approach into practice. It lists things that can be done to support participants, build an inclusive group and follow good practice in reminiscence work. If you are using the RYCT approach for one-to-one work, many of the same essentials apply, apart from those specific to group work.

THE RYCT PROGRAMME

Remembering Yesterday, Caring Today aims to make a difference to families living with dementia by providing a time and place where they can go together to enjoy memories of the past and perhaps forget for a moment the difficulties of the present. The leaders and volunteers involved in a group are sensitive to the ways that the project can help families to cope with dementia, taking account of their circumstances and needs. They can also suggest ideas for manageable activities that can be tried out at home or when visiting someone in care, and useful publications (e.g. Heathcote 2007).

Participating in an RYCT group can have different value for different people. For example, some carers have found that it helped to put the current strains into a longer perspective and this enabled them to keep going at difficult moments. Others have said they learnt new ways of coping by being with people in a similar situation. For some the most significant thing has been seeing a relative with severe dementia enjoying the sessions and participating more than they initially expected.

For many families being in a new social group and making new friends through sharing memories was particularly significant. Some have said how good it was to be part of a social group in which allowances were made for the effects of dementia, and found that it helped to combat feelings of isolation and loneliness arising from their experiences of social situations where people with dementia were not welcomed.

Working with family carers

One of the challenges for project teams is balancing the sometimes conflicting needs of family carers and people with dementia. Family carers can often behave in ways that undermine the well-being of relatives with dementia. For example, they may talk negatively about them within earshot, talk for them when they are able to say things for themselves, or emphasise how dementia makes them different and less capable than they were before. We need to take a person-centred approach to carers as well as people with dementia, recognising how hard it is when someone close and familiar changes, and can no longer contribute in the same way as before.

It is important to recognise and respect the real difficulties under which the family carers are labouring in their daily lives and to have realistic expectations of what they can do and how much they can change. It is also important to realise that 'put downs' from your nearest and dearest are not necessarily as undermining as those from other people. In most cases relationships between carers and people with dementia go back many years and we have to acknowledge that it can be hard to change patterns of behaviour and communication that are set firm. On the other hand, people have various ways of being and behaving with close family, for example there may be differences between the private and public sides of a relationship. When carers and those they care for are feeling depressed and exhausted, their interactions are more likely to be negative. When they are feeling happy and relaxed, we are more likely to see positive interactions.

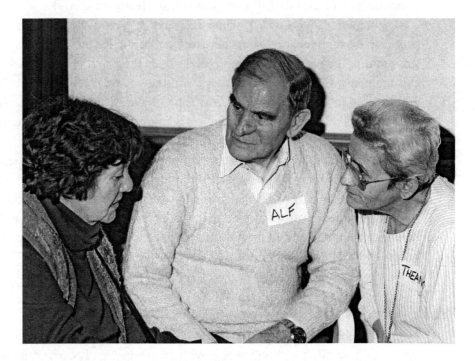

Figure 4.2: Alf and Theano enjoy talking as a couple with Doris

One of the strengths of the RYCT programme is to create an atmosphere in which carers can forget worry and despair, and become absorbed in the activities, at least for a short while. It is important that they experience the pleasure of reminiscing about their own lives so that they are not only in an enabling role during the sessions, and time and space must be made for this to happen. When they recall past times, they will often remember the feelings associated with those times and in many cases this helps them to see the person they care for in a more positive light. However, some family carers have an enormous need to talk about the difficulties of caring. In the original pilot projects more than half the sessions were split into separate groups for carers and people with dementia to accommodate this need. However, later groups have found that this is not always necessary, and that it can be better to take carers who need to relieve their feelings to one side for a one-to-one chat than to undermine the 'togetherness' of the programme by having a lot of split sessions. Splitting the group for a short period within selected sessions has proved to be a successful compromise. It provides an opportunity to explain the thinking behind the project to carers and to reinforce the importance of continuing reminiscence work in the home environment.

Carers are keen to learn useful strategies for coping from one another, and most are pleasantly surprised by what their person can still do and take a pride in helping that person to succeed. When project leaders and volunteers model positive and respectful approaches towards people with dementia, most carers are quick to appreciate that this is what is required in the group, and will nearly always act in this way towards participants with dementia from other families, even if old habits take over when relating to their own person. Many carers are keenly aware of the ways that people with dementia are treated as non-persons, and very relieved to find themselves in a group where this is not the norm. However, it can be galling for a family carer when he or she sees others eliciting far more animated responses from their person. We need to address these feelings and put them into some perspective, recognising the novelty value of other people, the pleasure of being in the 'social swim' and the inevitability of showing one's 'best side' in public more than in the privacy of home.

We need to appreciate the special contribution that family carers make in enabling their relative with dementia to participate. Their knowledge of their relative can be invaluable to adapting the activities to suit each individual, and for choosing the photos and objects to bring from home. Of course, for many people with dementia the presence of the carer is important to feeling secure in an unfamiliar place.

The problem of ending

The RYCT programme was originally designed as a series of 18 weekly meetings and, for practical reasons, this was later reduced to 12 sessions. However, it was soon clear that most participants did not want the group to finish, and monthly reunion sessions are now seen as an integral part of the project. Participants in the pilot groups (and those that followed) told us how much they valued being in a group that felt friendly and welcoming. It gave them a chance to do something enjoyable together, and had become an important part of their social life so they did not want it to come to an abrupt end.

Many groups have insisted on having follow-up sessions so that their new relationships within the group could be sustained. In London the participating families have formed a committee and become an organisation in their own right called the Reminiscence Reunion Club. The carers have been greatly empowered by this. They have raised funds and are applying for charitable status, all of which reflects their commitment to continuing the creative reminiscence work which they have enjoyed so much. They want to create an ongoing, lasting reminiscence reunion group.

COMMENTS FROM PARTICIPANTS, LEADERS AND VOLUNTEERS

To give a glimpse of what an RYCT project can be like, we have included some comments from participants, leaders and volunteers. We have collected comments made by a great many of the people who have participated in RYCT groups. Here are a few examples:

Participants (including family carers and people with dementia)

I would recommend this project very highly… The person I am caring for thoroughly enjoyed coming along, having an opportunity to connect with her past through the activities… This is really the best thing she has had since the dementia began. I have learned that using memory is a means of helping the person I care for to reconnect with her identity and I can use this in the long term… The monthly reunions will provide a way of continuing, and this will be very important for both of us… This is a life-line in what would otherwise be an extremely stressful and isolated struggle. (Michael Dash, carer)

I surprised myself being so knowledgeable about cooking pancakes and fairy cakes although I don't cook much myself. I have learned that other people have similar problems, such as my short-term memory. We have all become friends over the weeks. (Iris Goodman)

Something I learned was to let Mum live her life in the world she inhabits now... I don't wear myself out trying to keep everything 'normal'... Laughter is a great tonic... Mum and I have thoroughly enjoyed Tuesday afternoons and I have learned a lot about how to manage the situation we both find ourselves in. (Marilyn Upson, carer)

A new resolution: to let Mum answer if someone asks her a question, even if it takes a long time or the answer is inaccurate. (Jill Lawrence, carer)

The sessions with other carers were very good because I was mixing with others who have the same problems. (Charles Hall, carer)

As we are coming to the end of these weekly reminiscence meetings I would like to say how much I have enjoyed meeting you all and thank you for your friendship. I mean all of you, helpers as well. I felt shy at first of mixing with strangers and did not really want to come. But even after the first week I looked forward to the next Tuesday as I felt warm and welcome and we started to talk openly about our experiences. We laughed, talked about old films and sang songs from days gone by. These weeks have brought me out of myself, so I thank you all once again. It has been great. (Bill Parker)

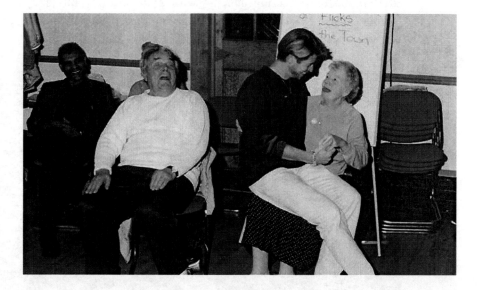

Figure 4.3: Bill has fun helping to recreate remembered movie moments, here singing 'Sonny Boy'

All the sessions were interesting and great fun. But I particularly liked the session on courtship and marriage, obviously a significant and well-remembered day for everyone. Funny too, with talk of reluctant bride-grooms and disagreeable mothers-in-law. (Kathleen Lynch, carer)

The session I enjoyed most was the dancing. It brought back memories. I liked everybody and made friends. (Joan Hall)

I learned that I have to wait for Peter to answer a question and not lose my temper. The project helped Peter to mix with other people and talk to them. (June Sweeney, carer)

I was surprised that I could get along so well with other people. I learned a lot about other people and how interesting they can be. (Claude Lemerle)

I remembered my childhood during the war times. People were friendly and their enthusiasm was contagious. I learned how to laugh again. (Ronald Hall)

I would recommend this project to a friend because they would like the way we carry on and get together. (Alice Richards)

I enjoyed the session on handling the babies because of remembering so far back. I was surprised that the wife adapted herself with regards to her memory. (Reg Richards, carer)

I enjoyed the session on jobs, reminding me of years ago when I was a hair-dresser, and remembering dancing with Zygmund (my husband) at the Winter Garden Blackpool. It was nice seeing myself on film and everyone was very friendly and talked to each other. (Amy Zadros)

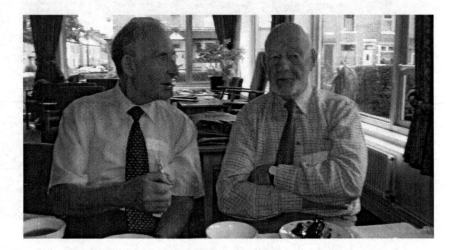

Figure 4.4: Peter and Jack, both ex-RAF, find plenty of memories in common

I go to a lot out of groups, but this is the one I like the best. (Charlie Green-wood)

I remembered putting the children to bed in the dark and leaving a candle burning for them. I want to forget sad memories. (Essielynne Locke)

I would recommend this project highly. I learned to encourage Mum to express herself and to give her time. It has not solved the problem of Mum remembering everything, but it has given her the confidence to at least try things first and think positive. Thank you. (Jennifer Locke, carer)

I'm sure I speak for a lot of family carers here when I say that we have really appreciated these reminiscence afternoons. I'm a different person com-pletely from when we first started meeting. I was a wreck. Now I feel I've got a lot of friends, everyone's friendly and I can talk to everybody here in the group. It's a great project. A marvellous thing. (John Pettit)

Comments from group leaders

This programme helps people value their lives and appreciate experiences of others through the rich human activity of reminiscing. Over eight years of co-leading RYCT groups, I have had the privilege of learning about the early lives and experiences of those with dementia and their carers. I am also more in touch with my own reminiscences, as we all contribute to the rich pool of life experiences in RYCT groups.

Sometimes my communication with a person with dementia has been only through their facial expressions and body language. Often through drawing – for example, a gentleman described his childhood home in Iraq to me, which I sketched. The more I questioned and clarified his memories, the more detail he provided. A real sense of his past was given and then shared with the whole group. Relationships between families, volunteers and workers evolve and deepen over the weeks because we enter into a process of revealing ourselves. (Caroline Baker)

More than anything, the success of the project lay in providing a time each week when everyone enjoyed the good and positive things about each other. For people with dementia there are few opportunities for enjoying a normal social occasion. The project helped this to happen. The telling and hearing of stories, the pleasure for both listener and teller, and the shared memories of objects and places provided a rich backdrop against which trust and relationships were built up. The use of reminiscence took the focus away from the present to times when both carers and people cared for were leading full and independent lives, reminding them of their self-worth and separate identities as individuals. The combination of reminiscence and the attention given to listening to one another was a powerful one for both carers and people with dementia. (Sarah Hodgson)

The benefits of participating in a programme of reminiscence to both those with dementia and their carers was palpable. The older people with memory difficulties grew in confidence as they discovered that they could still recall the distant past. They also rediscovered long forgotten skills. The carers, particularly family members, enjoyed learning new things about those they cared for and appreciated the techniques used in reminiscence to aid communication, which had all too often become difficult. The carers welcomed the opportunity to share their own recollections and the chance to mix with others who were facing similar difficulties. Many lasting friendships were formed. (Jean Valsler)

Travelling together into memories was a positive tool that none of the families had thought of using before joining the project. It was particularly effective for the people with dementia. They were the ones who had the greatest enthusiasm for seeking and finding their memories. They seized this opportunity for their own validation. They began to express their feelings more freely. It seemed that they had their place in the group and they took it. (Marie-Louise Carrette)

Day-to-day care routines emphasise the roles of carer and dependent, whereas reminiscence encourages family interaction which is close to normal. The simple pleasure of recognising a familiar object or recalling a forgotten melody were rays of sunshine in the fog of forgetfulness. Perhaps the feeling of pleasure enhanced their lives briefly, even if the reason for it was instantly forgotten. (Taina Johansson)

Comments from volunteers

Some of my most enjoyable memories of these weekly sessions are of when my own enthusiasms coincided with those of the person with dementia. The discovery of a shared knowledge of motorcycles with Alan, for example, formed the basis for a real connection. I would bring in bike parts like spark-plugs or chain sprockets, and Alan would handle these and scrutinise them intensely. It was clear, even without words, that these things brought back many memories of his life as a young man and the ambitious trips he had made (sometimes with his wife in the sidecar!) to other countries in Europe. If space and practicalities had not prevented it, I would have wanted to wheel in an old motorcycle for Alan. I know that if I myself were ever in his situation, I would find sharing an old passion like this with someone equally interested, an enjoyable and rejuvenating experience. (Alex Schweitzer)

It was a great experience to watch the husband's pleasure when his wife with dementia used the sewing machine and said, 'I was a seamstress long ago. I know this…' Another high point for me was when one of the ladies with dementia suddenly experienced something when she was given a piece of rock to handle while she simultaneously looked at a picture of a much-loved familiar mountain. I saw it in her face. She recognised the connection. (Norwegian volunteer)

I always left the sessions feeling better than I had done when I went in. I remember mentioning this in a debrief meeting, and everyone else felt the same. (Anne Haughie)

The project allows you to share memories with the person you are caring for and I found out things about Noel, my husband, that I didn't know before. I later became a volunteer on the project and it has helped me feel useful. Now I am there to support other families, but it helps that I understand what they are going through. When I first joined the project I was always shy

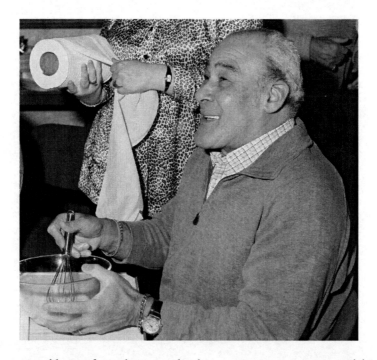

Figure 4.5: Noel having fun making pancakes during a Reminiscence Reunion Club cooking session

about doing things like role play. I always hoped I wouldn't be picked to join in, but now I have no problem with it. We've discussed so many topics and acted out so many different parts that I'm quite comfortable with it. In fact, I think it has made me a more confident person. Now I speak up more in meetings and I have become the co-chair of the Reminiscence Reunion Club. I've never done anything like that before and I'm proud of myself. (Jeanette Darrell)

Chapter 5

Organising a Reminiscence Project

In the RYCT projects, groups meet weekly for a two-hour session at the same time each week over a period of 12 weeks. Before holding the first session you will need to:

- recruit group leaders with appropriate experience
- recruit volunteers
- provide training and preparation for the project team
- recruit participants
- organise preliminary visits
- find a suitable venue
- organise transport to the venue
- produce written material (invitations to participants, handouts for volunteers, etc.)
- gather together equipment and resources
- plan debriefing, monitoring and evaluation
- set up monthly reunion sessions for when the weekly meetings come to an end.

RECRUITING THE PROJECT TEAM
Group leaders

You need two paid project workers to be group leaders or facilitators, preferably with reminiscence training and experience to organise the group and
lead sessions. Past project workers have included people from a wide range
of disciplines, including theatre workers, visual artists, drama therapists, occupational therapists, psychologists, historians, musicians and community
development workers. Group work skills are essential to the successful
running of RYCT groups, and facilitators with performance or teaching experience have been particularly effective in energising the families, encouraging them to take risks and to try out new approaches. In most cases, project
workers have worked together with someone whose skills differ from and
complement their own. All group leaders should also have some previous
experience of reminiscence and some understanding of the issues around
caring for someone with dementia.

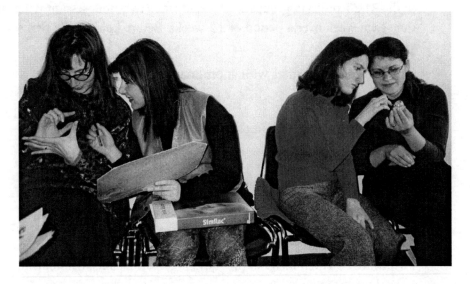

*Figure 5.1: Exploring non-verbal communication in a training workshop for group leaders in
Cluj, Romania starting reminiscence work with people with dementia*

Volunteers

You need to recruit volunteers who are enthusiastic about reminiscence,
happy to participate in the various creative approaches to developing memories (enactments, singing, etc.) and capable of working within the RYCT
ethos. You need sufficient volunteers to ensure that participants can have in-

dividual attention when they need it. If possible, have at least one volunteer per family. Past volunteers in RYCT projects have included Alzheimer's Society members, retired people, students, ex-carers, trainee arts workers, retired social workers and a taxi driver. In some RYCT projects health professionals wanting to learn more about reminiscence have joined as volunteers, seeing this as a valuable training opportunity. These have included occupational therapists, speech therapists, psychologists, nurses and care workers.

PREPARATION FOR THE PROJECT TEAM

Members of the project team, by which we mean group leaders, volunteers and anyone else who will be actively supporting the families through the project, need the following:

- direct experience of doing reminiscence by working with their own memories and participating in similar reminiscence activities to those that will be used in the RYCT group

- an opportunity to get to know more about one another's lives and particular skills through working together on reminiscence activities

- an insight into what it might feel like to have dementia and imagining how the world might look from the person with dementia's point of view

- some idea of the disabilities and difficulties that people with dementia are likely to experience

- an introduction to the experiences of family carers

- an introduction to positive approaches to people with dementia

- to know what to do and what to avoid when relating to people with dementia (e.g. utilising people's strengths and retained abilities, not testing them or exposing their limitations)

- to understand the essentials of the RYCT approach

- an opportunity to air worries and concerns about working with dementia and about how to handle situations that are likely to crop up during the project

- encouragement to play an active part in sessions, planning and evaluation.

Chapter 6 provides suggested training activities for the project team.

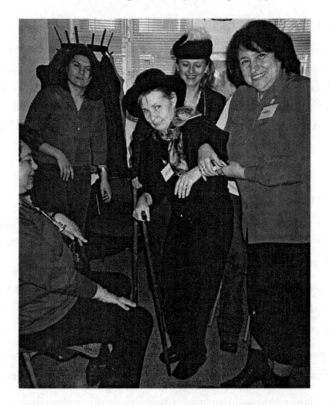

Figure 5.2: Trying out the improvisation approach in a training workshop in Sibiu, Romania, where workers explored their own memories before working with others

RECRUITING AND PREPARING PARTICIPANTS

Participants can come from a range of sources in the local area. These have included the following:

- Alzheimer's Society groups

- hospital memory clinics

- community psychiatric nurses involved in outreach work with families

- local doctors and medical surgeries

- via local newspaper advertisements

- via local newsletters

- via local respite care organisations such as Crossroads

- via local day centres.

You will need to think about the size of your group, bearing in mind the size of the room and the fact that most weeks some people will be absent. In the past RYCT groups have included anything from five to ten families. You need to recruit participants who will be able to cope with a group situation. Some people with hearing, visual or severe communication difficulties may find it hard to settle in a group, but we have found that some people with these difficulties have been able to enjoy the sessions and participate actively.

Home visits

It is important for members of the project team to visit each family before the group begins as it will help to prepare both participants and members of the project team.

The home visit is intended to:

- welcome the families to the project

- explain what will happen

- give reassurance – there are often worries about joining a new group

- discover something about the past and present lives of the families

- gain ideas about the reminiscence triggers that may be brought from home or referred to during the project.

When possible, this visit should be by two people, so that separate attention can be given to the person with dementia and to other family members. It is a good idea to involve volunteers in these visits and, where appropriate, use this as a basis for a continuing link between the family and a particular project worker or volunteer.

PRACTICAL MATTERS
Finding a suitable venue

Find a room with as many of the following features as possible:

- looks, or can be made to look, attractive

- good light and ventilation

- quiet and free from interruptions

- warm, comfortable and safe

- not too 'precious' a space, so some 'mess' can be made there during practical activities

- flexible seating so everyone can see and hear in the whole group and move easily into smaller groups

- convenient access to toilets

- somewhere to display memory triggers

- space to display products of the sessions

- enough room to move about, dance, perform improvisations

- disabled access

- facilities for making refreshments, and ideally for cooking activities

- use of a second room during sessions in which carers will meet separately for part of the time.

Arranging transport

Some participants may have cars, or family members who can drive them to meetings but, for those without, it is essential to provide transport that allows participants to attend without a great deal of effort and anxiety. Some can manage public transport, but for many a minibus, taxi or volunteer driver is the only practicable way to get to meetings.

Equipment and resources

You will need to organise appropriate resources and equipment for each session. Here is a list of essential and optional items:

Essential

- a suitable collection of objects to trigger memories appealing to all the senses, including hearing, smell, taste, touch as well as sight. These need not be expensive and can be gathered over a period from boot sales, junk shops and local collections. Relatives can be invited to help increase the stock of trigger items by loaning things from their own homes for the duration of the project

- small notebook, wallet folder or file for each family to use for record-keeping
- labels or badges for names
- camera
- paper, coloured pens, paint, scissors
- basic props such as work tools, kitchen and washing implements, hats, shawls, aprons
- food and drink
- CD or tape player.

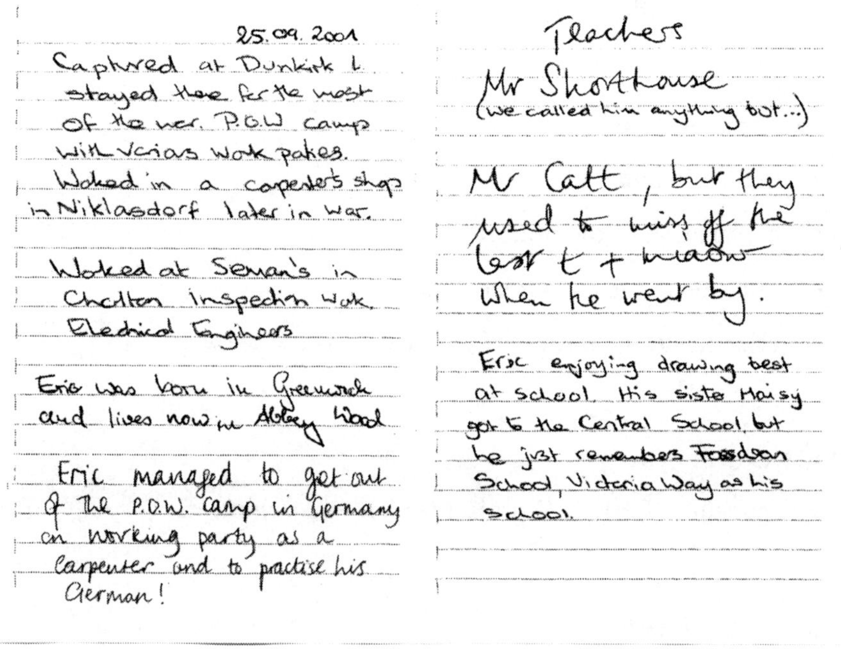
25.09.2001
Captured at Dunkirk & stayed there for the most of the war. P.O.W camp with various work parties. Worked in a carpenter's shop in Niklasdorf later in war.

Worked at Seman's in Charlton inspection work. Electrical Engineers

Eric was born in Greenwich and lives now in Abbey Wood

Eric managed to get out of the P.O.W. camp in Germany on working party as a carpenter and to practise his German!

Teachers
Mr Shorthouse
(we called him anything but...)

Mr Catt, but they used to miss off the last t + miaow when he went by.

Eric enjoying drawing best at school. His sister Maisy got to the Central School but he just remembers Fossdean School, Victoria Way as his school.

Figure 5.3: A page from Eric and Joan's notebook

Optional

- video camera and video or DVD player
- live music (piano, guitar or accordion) a great advantage, but not essential as the group can sing the songs they remember anyway.

Written material and handouts

You will need to provide various items of written material in the course of the project. You will find sample documents you can modify and handouts you can use in the Appendix, except where page numbers are given.

For everyone

- a timetable of the project including the topics to be covered (add dates to the list of sessions on p.127)
- the group agreements
- 'Hopes and fears' and 'Hopes and fears revisited' forms
- final evaluation form

For participants

- invitation letter
- explanation of the project
- introduction to the project team
- clearance form asking for permission to use photos

For the volunteers

- guidelines for RYCT project leaders and volunteers

For the group leaders

- general instructions for sessions (pp.104–9)
- attendance record
- session record – participants
- session notes
- following the RYCT approach – checklist

Planning for reunion sessions

You will need to plan ahead for reunion sessions on a monthly basis when the series of weekly meetings comes to an end. Transport, venue, and on-going facilitation and volunteer input will need to be organised. There is a list of suggested themes for reunion sessions at the end of Chapter 7.

MANAGING THE SESSIONS AND STRUCTURING THE PROJECT

General instructions for sessions

Preparation

- Prepare the room and equipment before each session. Select triggers and props carefully, drawing upon what the project team has found out about participants.

- Plan the seating carefully. Think about anxiety, especially in early sessions (e.g. people with dementia may need someone very attentive to support them if seated away from their relatives). Group people around common interests as they emerge, or blossoming friendships. Recognise the need for family carers to have a break and talk to each other when planning seating.

- Make sure that it is possible to switch between small and large group activities without needing to move too much furniture.

- For each theme, select from the suggested activities those which you think will work for your group. Be flexible and depart from the session plan if necessary. It is useful to build into the session an opportunity for the project workers to meet for a few minutes (perhaps during the tea-break) to revise plans as seems desirable.

- Provide a range of carefully chosen multi-sensory triggers appropriate to each theme (objects, images, music both live and recorded) and be sure to allow time for the people with dementia to respond to these triggers.

- In joint groups of people with dementia and their carers, plan to make time in some of the sessions (we suggest you do this in four of the following sessions – 3, 5, 7, 8, 9, 10) for the family carers to meet as a separate group. You will need the use of another room for this, or, if this is absolutely impossible, then a separate part of the main room. If possible, find an appropriate way (preferably related to the topic) to take the family carers into a separate group without too much disruption. Use this time with the carers to explain reminiscence and do some basic exercises to illustrate the principles of reminiscence, such as active listening, reflecting back what the person has said, and re-telling for that person what you know of his or her own life. (See 'Separate time for family carers' in Chapter 6.)

Managing sessions

- You can have one leader for the session, with the co-leader in a supporting role, or different members of the team can take the lead for different parts of the session, but make sure that everyone in the team is clear about their responsibilities.

- Use members of the project team to facilitate work in small groups.

- Manage feedback carefully so that it does not go on for too long. For example, use one person from each small group discussion to summarise and facilitate feedback from that group. The spokesperson should give prominence to the stories of the people with dementia and create opportunities for them to speak for themselves.

- When people have settled in, encourage family members to work with other participants, not exclusively with their own relative.

- Some people will finish exercises very quickly. In this case, check if they have fully understood the exercise and help them to explore it more deeply before suggesting that the whole group move on to the next activity.

- Round off sessions with a summary and appreciation of what has been done.

Checking on routine essentials

- Make sure that members of the team are available to give participants a warm welcome on arrival.

- Use name labels in every session – they can be a great help to people who find it hard to remember names.

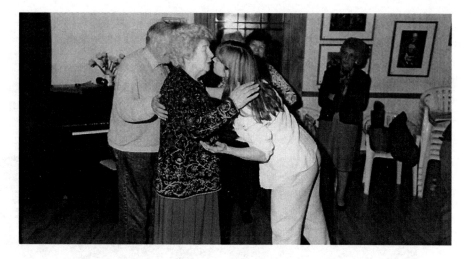

Figure 5.4: Greetings from the group leader on arrival at the session

- Ensure that everyone can see and hear in the large group, and adjust seating arrangements accordingly at the outset, and when the whole group re-forms after breaking into small groups.

- Organise record-keeping, providing notebooks, wallets, files or folders for each family. In joint groups, family members can take these home and use them to record reminiscence activities undertaken between sessions. Ask families to bring these in each week and give them time to share anything they have entered since the last session. When family carers are not involved it is best to keep the notebooks at the venue where the sessions take place. It is a good idea to provide some time for record-keeping during the sessions. Volunteers and group leaders can use the record books to write down interesting stories remembered by the people with dementia and activities they have been involved in during the session. When photos are taken of group activities or products, you can produce copies for participants to put in their record books.

- Give the family carers ideas for practical activities related to each session to do at home which will stimulate the person with dementia and relate to his or her known past interests. Suggest outings or visits to places connected with their past lives.

- Announce the content of the next session and encourage families to bring relevant items from home.

- Organise debriefing time for the project team to reflect together, evaluating each session, and noting individual responses.

- In the event of absence from the group, ensure that somebody contacts the family to check on their welfare, tell them about the theme for the next session and encourage their return to the group as soon as possible.

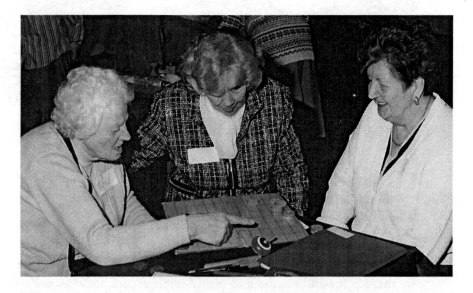

Figure 5.5: A game of draughts in the group stimulates memories and communication

Structuring the sessions

In all sessions, make sure that you have the following:

- reminiscence triggers offered to stimulate informal conversation relevant to the theme while the group gradually assembles

- an opening where participants are warmly welcomed and helped to tune in to what is happening. This can include a brief reminder of what happened in the last session

- warm-up exercises related to the theme; physical contact as appropriate

- main activities related to an agreed theme

- a closing where

    o the work of the session is summed up and appreciated

○ suggestions are made for work at home arising from the session, and participants are encouraged to think about the next session, including items they can bring in from home to help

○ good-byes are personal and appreciative.

You will almost certainly find that you do not have time for all the activities suggested in the outline plans. You can select or modify the suggested activities for each session to suit your group. If so, monitor what you keep in and leave out. Make sure that you:

• offer all the different creative elements during the 12 weeks: story-telling, improvisation, singing, dancing, mime, writing, practising old skills, drawing and cooking or gardening

• have at least one session where you create an environment that fits the theme (as in schooldays, courting and weddings)

• ensure that there is a balance between time spent in small groups and in the whole group

• use time in the whole group to celebrate and congratulate participants (e.g. make opportunities to present something to the whole group, such as re-posing wedding photos or re-enacting the presentation of prizes they won, as suggested in the schooldays session)

• make sure that everybody feels included, and that they have experiences and life stories to contribute. For example, in the session 'The next generation – babies and children,' participants may not have had children of their own, but looked after other people's children or worked with children. 'Holidays and travel': for some, the most significant memories of travel are not to do with holidays, but relate to wartime experiences, or travelling to a new country. If so, change the emphasis of the activities to reflect this.

DEBRIEFING, MONITORING AND EVALUATION

Schedule time at the end of each meeting, after the families have left, for the rest of the project team to reflect on the session. This is the best possible time to discuss issues that have arisen and make use of observations in planning the next session. To complete a record of what happened, photocopy the session record form in the Appendix and fill one in for each meeting,

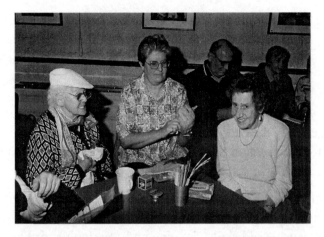

Figure 5.6a: Small group share winter memories

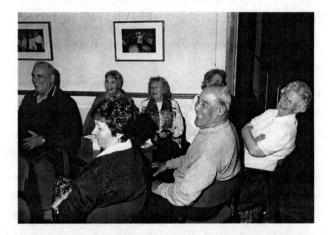

Figure 5.6b: Enjoying feedback of winter memories from other groups

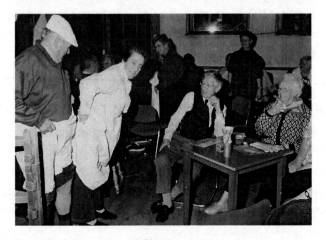

Figure 5.6c: Playing back the memories of keeping warm in winter

drawing upon everyone's observations and opinions. For sample session records see Chapter 7.

If some volunteers have to miss the debriefing meeting, for example due to giving participants lifts, you need to organise an alternative time for them to give feedback and contribute to planning.

Use the 'Adherence to project checklist' in the Appendix to monitor the project to ensure that you are including all the essential features of the RYCT programme. Video taken during sessions can be helpful in judging whether you have included all the essential features and it can also be helpful to have someone in the role of observer during some or all of the sessions who can feed back on what he or she has observed. Monitoring in this way is good practice and helps the team to meet the needs of all participants. (See Chapter 3 for a discussion of using evaluation to learn from experience.)

Training for the Project Team and Family Carers

TRAINING ACTIVITIES FOR THE PROJECT TEAM

Some of the exercises specified below for training the project team are also suggested for use when training family carers and they are described in greater detail later in this chapter.

Understanding how people experience dementia

- Invite team members to participate in listening and not listening exercises and to reflect on what both feel like. (See pp.117–120 later in this chapter for a full description of this and the next three exercises.)

- Experience what it is like to be talked about and talked over, which is the experience of many people with dementia, through an exercise in a group of three, where each takes it in turn to be the person who is excluded.

- Experience what it is like to find difficulty in locating the right form of words by counting to ten before joining in the conversation and seeing how it has moved on before you can catch up with it.

- Experience what it is like not to be able to speak but still to have things you wish to communicate, such as a message, a memory or a wish.

Experiencing reminiscence

- Choose a subject (e.g. a childhood friend, or leaving school) and ask the group to work in pairs. Within the pairs, take it in turns to speak, each partner taking three minutes to speak while the other listens. The listener should try to remember what his or her partner said so he or she can report on it.

- Ask the pairs to join with another pair to make a group of four. Ask each person to tell his or her partner's story and to check with the original teller, thus confirming his or her ownership of the story.

- As a whole group, discuss what it felt like to do this. Explore questions such as:

   o What did it feel like to share a personal memory and listen to the partner's memories?

   o Did you find some common ground?

   o What was it like to have a personal memory shared with the wider group?

   o How did it feel to have someone tell your story for you?

- Returning to the same groups of four, ask each group to choose one of the stories they have shared and make a short scene out of it to play to the wider group. Only allow eight to ten minutes for them to prepare these scenes, as the idea is to improvise spontaneously rather than to produce a polished performance.

- As a whole group reflect on the experience of dramatising the stories, with questions such as:

   o Have you enjoyed hearing about very different lives?

   o How did it feel if your story was chosen/not chosen?

   o What was it like to be part of the scene?

   o Did you enjoy watching the other scenes?

- Give the group the experience of using objects to trigger memories. Use objects appropriate to the age-group of the people being trained. Arrange the objects on a table and invite every person to choose something which 'calls out to them'. Invite a few people to tell the rest of the group why they have chosen that object. Draw a picture to

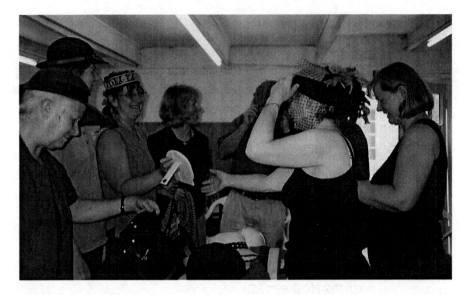

Figure 6.1: A practical training day for RYCT workers and volunteers

explain the memories associated with the object and write a caption underneath. Allow only eight to ten minutes for this exercise. Make a small 'exhibition' of the drawings and visit one another's exhibits.

- Ask the group for suggestions of songs that capture the themes which have emerged from these exercises. Sing them together and see if, by pooling memories, you can remember all the words.

Working together and becoming an effective reminiscence team

- Choose a theme and brainstorm as a group how it could be explored with participants with dementia. Include objects which might trigger memories (and where to locate them), images and relevant songs linked to the theme. Now go to the relevant session description in the manual and look through the proposed structured exercises. Decide what each person in the team can contribute to the session, including refreshments, time-keeping, ensuring that people with dementia are not left alone, supporting people who seem distressed.

- Give the trainees an opportunity to experience a whole-group improvisation, so they can participate effectively when this strategy is used with people with dementia. Choose subjects such as schooldays, going to the cinema or a wedding and spontaneously play out a familiar situation, making sure everybody has a role to play. Use examples from Session plans 3, 5 and 6 in Chapter 7 to guide you here. Discuss how the exercise went and any further ideas for ensuring that the people with dementia have a good time.

- Discuss the importance of post-session debriefing as a way to continue to build the team and consider how to ensure that all members of the team can contribute their feedback if they have to leave as soon as the session is over.

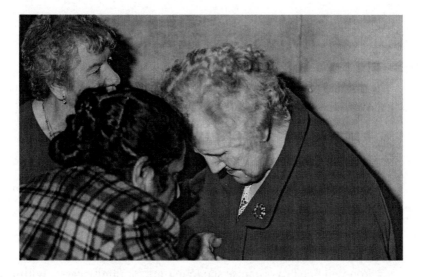

Figure 6.2: Afrose, a community psychiatric nurse working with the RYCT project in London, is quick to respond to Doris's temporary distress

Airing worries and concerns

- Make time for people to express any worries or concerns they have about working with people who have dementia.

- Discuss how the team will handle anything that people are worried about, and situations that often crop up in RYCT projects.

- Relate these discussions to the essential ways of working, and make sure that everyone has a copy of the handout 'Guidelines for RYCT project leaders and volunteers' (see Appendix).

There should be some discussion concerning situations that often crop up and that the team may need to handle:

- people with dementia being anxious or distressed
- carers being distressed
- carers correcting their relative
- carers who speak for their relative
- carers talking negatively in front of their relative
- people wanting to leave
- people not arriving for the group.

TRAINING ACTIVITIES FOR FAMILY CARERS
Separate time for family carers

The training for family carers is informal in style and takes the form of practical exercises designed to:

- raise consciousness about positive approaches to caring
- increase awareness about reminiscence
- demonstrate how the reminiscence activities in the group can be continued at home.

The four outline sessions suggested here include exercises designed to cover each point.

You will need to organise separate time for family carers within some of the sessions in order to explain reminiscence to them and help them to see how they can help their person with dementia within the sessions and at home.

In these sessions, the family carers will leave the joint group for 45 minutes to one hour and meet in a separate space, preferably another room. You need to arrange this to cause as little upset as possible for the participants with dementia, and to make it fit naturally into the sessions, finding a good moment for them to return and see what has been done in their absence. If it is possible to meet family members before the group starts to explain the project, this can be an advantage. Otherwise it is probably wise to wait until Session 3 to divide the group, so that everyone has had time to settle in and the people with dementia will be less worried about being left.

N.B. You may find that some families do not wish to separate and prefer to stay together throughout the project, maximising their shared enjoyment. If this is the case, project workers and volunteers should respect their wishes, but ensure that they offer strong models of the teaching points contained in the training exercises which follow. You may find that it works to take carers in small groups of two to four into a separate room for shorter periods throughout the project in order to do these exercises. The following sessions lend themselves to dividing the group:

- Session 3: Schooldays

- Session 5: Going out and having fun

- Session 7: Homes, gardens and animals

- Session 8: The next generation – babies and children

- Session 10: Holidays and travel

Outline plans for four sessions with family carers

Carers' Group 1: About reminiscence and active listening

Objectives

- To find out how carers and those they care for are feeling about the project.

- To explain why reminiscence is a helpful activity for people with memory problems.

- To demonstrate some of the do's and don'ts of reminiscence.

- To convey the RYCT ethos.

- To give carers an opportunity to say something about the home situation, if they feel a need to do so.

Outline plan

1. Listening and not listening

Ask people to work in pairs and tell each other about how they spent last Sunday. Take it in turns to speak, but do not listen to one another. In fact, make it clear that you are preoccupied and haven't really got the time or inclination to listen. See how long the person speaking can carry on in the face of this indifference. Ask the group to consider what it feels like not to be listened to and to share how often they find themselves too rushed or tired to listen to their person.

Then try what the opposite response feels like. Try exchanging memories of what Sundays were like in childhood. Take it in turn to speak in the pair, but this time show you are interested by your body language, by asking additional questions, by keeping some eye contact.

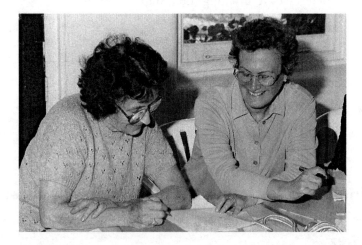

Figure 6.3: Madeline Armstrong, group leader, helps Vi, a family carer, to remember and record stories about her own childhood

Ask the group to reflect on how they might try checking on themselves at home to see if they can make time in the day for some 'active listening' as in the last exercise.

2. Speaking for another person

Ask participants to join another pair to make a four. Everyone tells the other three people the story they have just heard from their partner (or as much of it as they can remember) about childhood Sundays. This exercise tests how effectively people have listened to one another and how much they have retained. It also gives participants the opportunity to experience the positive and negative aspects of having someone else speak for you and tell your story.

3. Being outpaced: experiencing what it is like not to find the words in time

Arrange people in threes and ask two of them to discuss favourite places they have been on summer holidays or a holiday they are planning to take. Ask the third person to count to ten before joining in with his or her comments. Usually the conversation will have moved on and that person will be made to feel redundant. The 'slower' person should feed back to the others what this feels like and then change roles so that everyone experiences the situation. Offer the suggestion that carers try out counting to ten before speaking for their person. They can report back to the next carers' session about whether this makes a difference.

4. Speaking over someone

In a variant of this exercise, two people talk to each other about the third in his or her presence, discussing what he or she likes, or the things he or she 'gets up to' and what it is like to care for him or her. The 'cared for' person remains silent. If he or she attempts to join in, he or she is excluded by the others. The 'outsiders' should have an opportunity to give feedback on what this feels like, and others can swap positions so they too can be on the receiving end of what are very common experiences for people with dementia. Suggest that carers monitor the occasions on which they speak about their relative in their presence and also note how often their comments are negative.

John Goodman, a family carer, kept a diary of the RYCT project. This is his record of one of the sessions for carers.

An extract from John Goodman's diary

Pam and Adrian had a chat to all of us and the theme was that carers should give their folks the chance to answer when spoken to and not jump in with the answer. I must admit I am guilty of this.

We then did an exercise in groups of three where one was the person with impaired memory, who had to count to ten before answering, one had to ask questions, and the third person to answer. I think this brought home to us carers what we do wrong with the best of intentions to our loved ones. We must let our loved ones speak for themselves and listen to their answers.

Then we came to a very good exercise of which not only us carers but many hospital staff are guilty. In this exercise two of us talked about the third member as if they were not present. When it came your turn to be the one that was being spoken about, even though it was pretend, it really brought it home to me what it feels like. We must not do this. We must always give them the chance to speak for themselves whenever possible.

We also did an exercise where we told something to another person in the group and they told our story for us. That was quite a nice feeling because you knew the other person had listened to you. Pam and Adrian told us that our loved ones would probably enjoy hearing their history repeated by us, provided we ensured that they could join in and feel part of it. This was a very good session and I think that all the carers could see which way we were being led. I think this will help us all.

N.B. Extracts from John's diary have been used in a theatre production by Pam Schweitzer entitled *Stories*, featuring the voices of people with dementia and family carers, which plays at conferences and training sessions to help raise consciousness amongst carers.

Carers' Group 2: About helping people with dementia to communicate

Objectives

- To explore the experience of dementia, especially communication difficulties.

- To raise awareness about the frustrations experienced by people with dementia.

- To encourage carers to take time to try to understand what their relative is trying to say.

- To exchange ideas about ways of keeping communication going at home.

Outline plan

1. Feedback from carers

Allow some time for carers to talk about if and how they have been using the ideas of the project at home. Have they found that 'active listening' and 'counting to ten' have made a difference?

2. Incomplete communication

Although people with dementia may be able to speak fluently, it is sometimes difficult to understand exactly what they are getting at. It is important to try to understand or unravel what is being said. Ask the carers to consider the idea that they sometimes have to operate as though they are detectives working on an important case.

Ask people to work in groups of three or four and take it in turns to try to share a memory of a childhood illness or an accident, using only four words, and not necessarily the essential words. The others must try to fathom what happened.

Ask people to work in groups of three or four (with the same people as in the previous exercise or in a new grouping) and take it in turns to try explaining to the others about a special occasion from the past or a wish for the future *without using words at all*. The listeners have to guess what the other person is trying to tell them. After these two exercises, discuss the feelings of all parties and how they express their frustration.

3. Mystery moments

Ask carers to give examples of 'mystery moments' when they have not understood what the person they are caring for was trying to say to them or where both have become frustrated by their failure to communicate. Share experience and ideas in the group about how to be encouraging and patient in this mutually frustrating situation.

4. Responding positively

Indicate to carers that their person will have been involved in an activity without them while this separate session has been going on. Encourage and model a positive response to what the group and individuals within it have been doing in the carers' absence and what, if anything they have produced to share. If there are drawings or other products, invite carers to take them home and display them somewhere as a reminder of the group they now belong to.

A further extract from John Goodman's diary

On rejoining our loved ones, Iris came to me and said 'What did you do?' I immediately put my new knowledge to good use and said 'Let me know your side first and tell me what you have been up to.' Iris said she had played hopscotch and cricket with a wooden spade and a small ball, but she said they didn't have stumps, then went on to say they played marbles. I then said 'What else have you been doing?' Her remark was 'That's enough, ain't it?'

Carers' Group 3: Reminiscence at home
Objectives

- To encourage positive approaches to people with dementia and recognition of the efforts they may make to help with tasks at home.

- To enable the carers to support one another by exchanging good ideas.

- To raise awareness of small ways to make a difference to quality of life and sense of well-being of people with dementia at home.

- To offer ways of including reminiscence in daily life at home.

Outline plan

1. Feedback from the carers

Check with them whether they have modified any of their behaviour or attitudes as a result of what they have seen/heard in the sessions, and whether the adaptation helped.

How are their listening skills developing? Have they worn their 'detective hats' at all and have they understood any more of what their relative says, wants or needs as a result?

2. Praise and thanks

Ask the carers to tell one another about something their person still does around the house, such as washing up, making tea, digging the garden, or laying the table. Ask them to tell about how they respond to what their person does and what impact this might have. Compare this with how they might respond to the efforts of a grandchild and see if they can see alternative ways of reacting which might improve their person's confidence. Encourage the view that these efforts, even though they may be frustrating for the carer, need to be acknowledged and appreciated. They can help to reinforce their person's memories of themselves as 'doers', as active members of the family and community, still with something to contribute.

3. Including reminiscence in daily life

Suggest simple ways of including reminiscence in daily routines:

- Selecting suitable programmes on radio and TV in *Radio Times* and listening to or watching them together.

- Going on a visit to a remembered spot.

- Getting out old photo albums, going through them and adding captions as memories arise.

- Playing favourite music on CDs, tapes or records.

- Reading aloud a favourite novel or extracts from the newspaper.

- Putting souvenirs from holidays on a table and remembering those times together.

- Getting old work certificates or equipment out and recalling working days.

- Going to a boot fair or fete and buying items connected with the past.

4. Multi-sensory stimulus

Check also on whether carers are stimulating all their person's senses or over-relying on verbal communication. Suggest having the following handy:

- bags or small collections of objects to handle and sort through

- fabrics to feel and fold

- pots of herbs or medicines to smell

- raw ingredients to prepare and taste

- favourite music to listen to.

Suggest that the carers build into their everyday activities and routines opportunities for sensory stimulation and remembering. For example, when preparing food, encourage the person with dementia to handle and smell the ingredients and summon up past memories of cooking and eating.

Where the carer has to leave the person with dementia alone for a while, suggest that they leave interesting objects in the rooms the person is likely to visit. These can be photos or mementos laid out on a bed or coffee table, scarves to handle, a rummage box of old sewing things to sort out, an old school report or even a wedding telegram. Creating a trail in this way can give the person interesting encounters with the past through sensory stimuli, and the experience can be talked over together on the carer's return.

Encourage the completion of the scrap-books or notebooks supplied by the project with images and words from daily life at home as well as with records of what happened during the RYCT sessions and help them with this task, so that it is a joint undertaking.

5. The 'home team' working together

Emphasise the importance of doing these reminiscence activities jointly (not as a memory test) and allowing themselves, the carers, to find some enjoyment and satisfaction by sharing their own memories. Suggest that their person will probably respond to the positive atmosphere and sense of inclusion, even if unable to recall the memories for themselves. Recognising and appreciating the carers' memories (especially of things they have done together) can be pleasurable for people with dementia and increase their sense of themselves and their relationships.

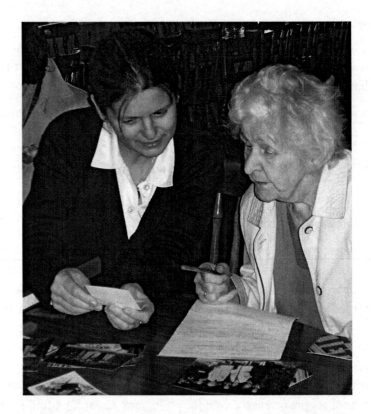

Figure 6.4: Looking at old family photos to jog memories in the Bangor RYCT project

Putting new ideas into practice at home: more from John Goodman's diary

Since the early days of Iris and me attending the reminiscence sessions, we have come a long way. Iris has always liked her holidays and I decided to give her those holidays that we missed when she was in hospital. I started by letting her sort out where she wanted to go. Before Iris went to hospital, she was always in charge of packing the two suitcases. She always did this with lists of all the things she would be packing and I had kept these lists. She got them out and spent a long time trying to make sense of them, but I stayed out of it. Slowly, very slowly, she sorted out everything we would need for our holiday in Wales, ironed and packed it and didn't forget anything. She also managed to repack the cases for our return, including the presents we had brought and nothing was broken. She also used the route map I had got for the journey. I knew the route, but with a little patience Iris did the navigation and she now does it without any help from me. If I had not had some training on the reminiscence project, I would have done all this myself.

I think I should say a little about how Iris spends her time when I go to work. As I said, when she first came out of hospital I could not leave her alone so my young sister stayed with her. Iris has always liked flowers and plants. At present she is starting to collect china 'double-boot' plant pots and plant them with very small leafy plants. I am sure they will grow given time.

Carers' Group 4: Using what they have learned on the project

Objectives

- To explore how the carers are using what they have learned on the project.

- To hear from the carers about new activities or changes they have made to the way they spend time at home.

- To exchange ideas about what works.

- To plan for the final session (see information below).

- To discuss the organisation and arrangements for a reunion group.

Outline plan

1. Discussion of reminiscence at home

Invite each carer to tell about one reminiscence-related action or activity they have tried at home and how it worked or did not work. Encourage exchange of ideas between carers about approaches they have found worthwhile and how their relative has reacted.

2. Preparing for the final session

Ask each family to prepare one or both of the following things to present at the final session:

- A short appreciation of their relatives, thinking about what is special and distinct about the life they have led, their special gifts and achievements in the past, and the good qualities they still have. Ask them to bring along one or two significant objects or documents connected to their relatives' past interests, achievements or activities.

- An account of a memorable event, activity or occasion they have experienced together, recently or a long time ago. Offer the suggestion that this activity is prepared jointly at home, or that it is prepared by the carer as a surprise for his or her relative. Some people will want to write something down, but most will probably prefer to talk 'off the cuff' about their person.

3. Monthly reunion sessions

Discuss with the carers whether they would like to participate in a monthly reunion group if it proved possible to organise this. Find out how they feel about extending the project in this way and what they would hope to gain from further sessions. This might be an opportunity to discuss with the carers how much additional responsibility they would be prepared to take in planning the sessions, preparing items to bring along, or even taking a role in leading part of a session.

A final extract from John Goodman's diary

Some months after joining the group, I took Iris back to the hospital with some chocolates for the staff who had looked after her during her stay. Of course all the questions were directed at me, but I didn't answer so Iris stepped in to do all the talking. Iris then went off happily with a nurse to chat with people she knew when she was in the ward. This showed me that, if given the chance, our loved ones will chat, but they will need more time... It's like a delayed reaction and that's why it really helps me now to count to ten before I answer for Iris.

Chapter 7

Reminiscence Sessions

Retracing the Life Course

OUTLINE TIMETABLE

The sessions are based on key stages in life which most people will have experienced and which will include everyone in the group. The chronological approach can also help families to take a longer view of their lives and undertake an informal 'life review' during these 12 weeks. You may need to modify the outline plans to fit your own situation. In doing this it is important to maintain the essential elements of the RYCT approach.

1. Introductions

2. Childhood and family life

3. Schooldays

4. Starting work and working lives

5. Going out and having fun

6. Weddings

7. Homes, gardens and animals

8. The next generation – babies and children

9. Food and cooking

10. Holidays and travel

11. Celebration

12. Rounding up and evaluation

Each session plan includes more activities than can be fitted into a single session. They are offered on the understanding that group leaders will design their own sessions choosing from the suggested activities. It is important to offer a range of activities to engage as many people as possible and achieve a balanced programme, as discussed in the previous chapter.

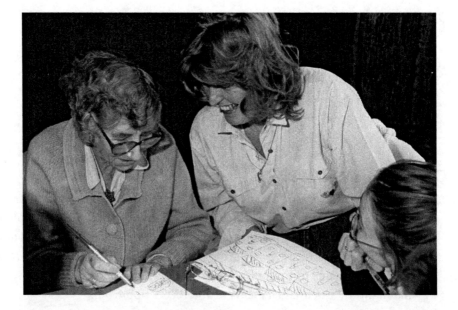

Figure 7.1: Edith remembers the mining village where she grew up and is prompted in this by Carol's questions. For some people drawing is an easier way to explore memories than talking about them.

Each outline session plan includes a sample set of group leader's notes, based on notes made by actual project leaders, showing what activities were used and what issues emerged, and giving a flavour of how the session went. (Many thanks to Caroline Baker whose notes provided the main source. Please note that participants' names have been changed to preserve anonymity.)

SESSION 1: INTRODUCTIONS
Objectives

- To make people feel welcome and at ease.
- To introduce people to each other.

- To get started on reminiscence.

- To generate interest and enthusiasm.

Outline plan

Triggers

- birth and marriage certificates, maps of the local area

- name books (for parents of new babies)

Opening

Welcome each family as they arrive and thank them for making the effort to come. Show new arrivals to seats, preferably at small tables with two families to a table, but at larger tables of eight or ten if necessary, with a team member assigned to work with them. Team members and volunteers make sure that everyone has a name label and encourage informal conversation. This is a possible moment to ask family carers who arrive early to complete their 'Hopes and fears' sheet (see Appendix) if they have not done so before. Otherwise, they can take the form home with them and bring it in the following week. When the group has assembled, the group leader calls everyone to turn their chairs around so they can see her or him or make a circle. The leader welcomes everyone to the group and announces that they will be meeting every week for 12 weeks, during which time he or she hopes they will all get to know one another, make friends, explore some memories and have fun. He or she suggests starting with an exercise.

Warm-up

Each person says their name and one thing they like. It is helpful to give a couple of examples first, such as walking, shopping, eating chips, seeing grandchildren, sleeping or listening to music. Give people a moment to prepare with the person sitting next to them, so that if someone is having difficulty with this there is help from a carer or volunteer to hand. Then go round the group, hearing each person, with the leader repeating what has been said and making connections, where they exist, with others in the group with similar likes. This exercise helps people to remember names and link them to people by association, for example 'I'm Mary and I like pear drops.'

Main activities

1. In small groups at each table, exchange information about their names. The team member facilitates, so that each person speaks in turn, and time is given to allow people who are slow to express themselves. Find out about the following (you could prepare a sheet for each group):

    *   names – first, middle and last

    *   where names came from, who chose them

    *   family history of name

    *   any local or national or international associations/links

    *   nicknames

    *   different names for different times and places, such as how you were known at home and at work, as a child or as an adult

    *   changes of name, for example, maiden name, married name, name on divorce, name used when in another country

    *   how people feel about their names

    *   if I could have chosen my own name…?

    *   anything else people want to say about their name.

    Feed back to the whole group what has emerged at each table. Project team can use this as an opportunity to make connections between people as the feedback is going on.

2. Invite everyone to get up and greet as many people as possible in the room, saying their own name and using lots of different ways of saying hello (saluting, bowing, shaking hands, waving, hugging, hand-slapping, thumbs up). The facilitator can start this off by demonstrating some of these. He or she should pick up connections between participants as they greet one another, such as ex-servicemen sharing a salute, ex-Brownies, Girl Guides and Scouts signalling one another, greetings associated with particular countries where participants have lived, and old-fashioned greetings like bows and curtseys, hat-tipping exchanged between participants.

Tea break: Serve tea and snack at group tables.

3. In the same small groups discuss where members grew up.

    *   What was the area like?

- Was it in a city, a town, or a village?

- Was it a flat, a house, a caravan?

- Was it cold or warm, tidy or a mess?

Take note of anything people want to say about where they grew up. Feed this back to the whole group.

4. Leader invites anyone who can remember to tell the group his or her childhood address.

5. Leader suggests that the names of the places where people grew up are recorded on a large piece of paper. During feedback leader and project team pick up and comment on any connections between group members.

6. Ask people to think of any song they can remember associated with the period in their lives or the place they have been remembering. Find a song which most people in the group can sing together.

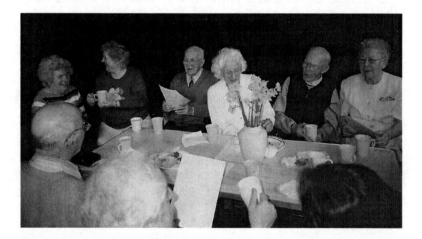

Figure 7.2: Tea-time for informal socialising followed by a short sing-song with piano accompaniment

Closing

Leader gives a summary to the whole group of what has been done during the session. In small groups, each family is given a pack about the project to take home. The plan for the following week is explained to the whole group. Everyone is asked to bring one or two photographs of themselves when young, and/or one or two objects associated with their childhoods. Thank people for coming and say good-bye to each person.

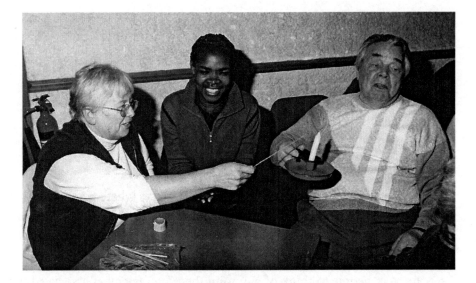

Figure 7.3: Bill remembers having a candle to light him to bed

---

Session notes: Introductions

Activities used today

- Introductions and name labels.
- Everyone said their names and something they enjoyed or liked.
- We repeated some of the things enjoyed, inviting the group to remember others.
- In small groups – talked about meaning, origin, feelings about names.
- Fed back to whole group.
- Greetings – naval, army, formal, friends, etc. across the room.
- Tea and share info about early origins, places.
- Fed back to whole group, writing places and names on a large piece of paper.
- Songs sung together – finished with 'We'll meet again'.
- Asked people to bring photos, certificates, objects to the next session.

Comments (what went well, what went not so well, who enjoyed what)

- All were willing to share information and memories in small groups.

- Almost everyone managed to contribute when going round the circle, a few were nervous (e.g. Max and Nell).

- In the large group we need to move around swiftly because of concentration levels and size of group. Volunteers need reminding to keep their stories brief.

- When reporting back from small groups, we must limit it to two comments/memories from each group, or attention wanes. Contributions should be acknowledged and valued in the small groups already.

- They were all happy to get up and interact physically and verbally, some members need this physicality regularly throughout session, (e.g. Fred and James).

Points to consider in future sessions

- Non-verbal methods of working are essential.

- Nell – try not to move her, triggers toilet needs.

- Meg – find best position for hearing.

- Collect 'Hopes and fears' sheet next time, have extra copies available.

SESSION 2: CHILDHOOD AND FAMILY LIFE
Objectives

- To develop the sense of belonging to the group.

- To introduce creative activities related to memory.

- To re-experience the feel of childhood.

- To work co-operatively to recall the past.

Outline plan
Triggers

- family photos

- family bible

- a sample family tree

- childhood games, skipping rope, conkers

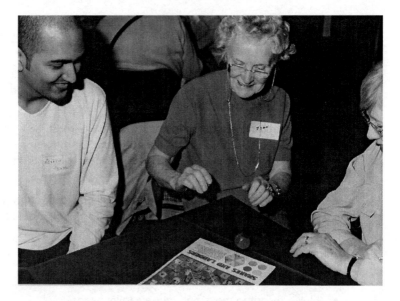

Figure 7.4: Joan enjoys a game of Snakes and Ladders with volunteers

(If you have people who grew up in other parts of the world, try to find appropriate objects to trigger their childhood memories.)

Opening

Members of the team welcome each family as they arrive and thank them for making the effort to come.

As they greet people, refer back to something they learned about them in the first week such as a special nickname, the place they came from, a bit of a song or something they liked.

Seat people at small tables (preferably two families to a table) in combinations which will maximise any common ground which emerged in the first session. Assign appropriate team members to each group. Team members give out name labels.

Warm-up

Working in the small groups, invite people to share the photos or objects they have brought in. Have some photos of babies and children or miscellaneous reminiscence objects to hand in case anyone has forgotten to bring their own. Team members can share their own photos and objects, but should be careful not to take too much time.

The team should encourage people with dementia to speak for themselves and address much of the conversation to them, leaving plenty of time for responses and not hurrying them. If possible, it is desirable to have a separate listener for each family member, so that carers can enjoy reminiscence at their own speed, and perhaps catch a glimpse of their relative engaging directly in exchange with someone else.

Main activities

1. Still in the small groups, team members ask participants to recall a family member or neighbour who was very important to them in their early years. This could be a grandparent, aunt or uncle, next-door neighbour, nanny or a brother or sister. Ask about what they were like. Draw a picture of how that person is remembered by the participant, including what they wore, their hair, what they might have been doing, their habits, behaviour, their quirks and what they commonly said.

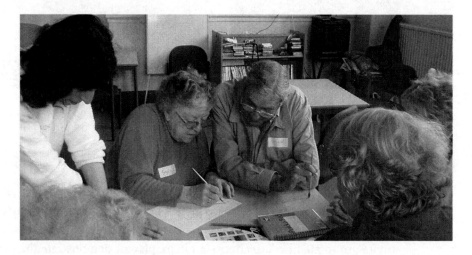

Figure 7.5: A volunteer and a participant draw a family memory together

An option here is to help draw a 'family tree' for the participants with dementia, with the help of their family members, featuring their most strongly remembered relatives.

Leader invites feedback from small groups to the whole group. Pictures, stories and family trees are presented and explained, and common ground highlighted (e.g. close relationship with a grandmother).

2. In small groups: each person (team members included) chooses one photo or object to go into a temporary group collage or 'exhibition of childhood' to be laid out on a large table. The leader invites each person to find a place for their photo or object in the 'Exhibition', which can be laid out on a table or even on the floor in the middle of the group, with or without accompanying captions. The leader invites people to explain the item they are contributing, with the help of a team or family member. Take a photo of this as a record of the group at work. Invite people to get up and look at the exhibition while tea is served.

Tea break: Serve tea and snack at group tables. During the tea-break put out a display of childhood games.

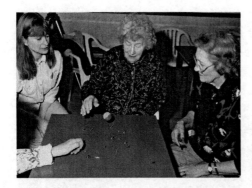 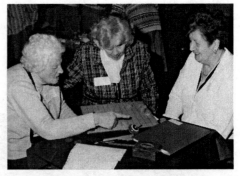

Figure 7.6: Amy enjoys a game of jacks   *Figure 7.7: A game of draughts in progress*

3. Childhood games

   Arrange a display of childhood games, marbles, balls, yo-yos, jacks, cards, skipping ropes, ludo, board games, cigarette cards or anything else you can find. (Use reproductions and modern versions where necessary.) Invite group members to choose an item, play or demonstrate the game and share memories with others. This may be an opportunity for mixing and making new connections with other people. Encourage participants to play the games with each other, moving around as necessary.

   Leader can invite members to show the rest of the group how the games were played and to share their memories about playing games (rules, cheating, winning, losing, etc.).

4. Ask the whole group if there are any songs associated with childhood games, including skipping and counting rhymes or songs connected

with the people everyone has been remembering. See if there is one that the whole group would like to sing.

Closing

Leader summarises what has been done.

Leader announces the theme for the following week and asks everyone to bring in any school reports they have held on to, any prizes, cups or trophies, photographs or objects associated with their schooldays, and their friends from that time or images of the area where they went to school.

Leader and team members remind everyone about their memory diaries and suggest that people write down some of the memories stirred by the session if they would like to.

Leader thanks everyone for coming. Personal good-byes to everyone.

Session notes: Childhood and family life

Activities used today

- Small tables arranged with images of childhood for people to look at as they arrived.

- In the whole group – recalled things they said they liked from previous week, introduced new people who were not at first session.

- In small groups recalled friends played with and games played. Summary versions relayed to wider group. Took a long time, but everyone joined in.

- Olive played childhood songs medley on piano and group mimed physical actions of remembered games. Everyone did this at same time, so no embarrassment.

- Posed the question: 'Who called you indoors for tea?' Moved into small groups to discuss inside environments and people who were there for them at home.

- During tea continued sharing memories of important people in childhood and at home.

- After tea, put board games, marbles, dominos, dolls, etc. on tables, triggering reminiscences on indoor play.

- Shared photos brought in by families.

Comments

- Did not get to drawing important people or family trees.

- Group very good at listening to each other in whole group.

- Commonalities and shared experiences greeted with pleasure.

- Observed people learning from each other how to support those with dementia: holding back, allowing their relative to speak, waiting, including.

- We allowed time to settle into the group and adjust to the space when they arrive. Perhaps try themed music on piano as people arrive and greet one another.

- Adequate balance of physical activity/verbally based activities.

Points to consider in future sessions

- Making real greetings and organising seating an important part of session.

- Allowing time for volunteers to have briefing before session.

- Try different combinations of couples and separating some of the couples.

- Carers' separate session next session will go some way to shaking up seating.

- Volunteers to place themselves between couples to maximise their expertise.

- Lucy (student occupational therapist (OT)) is willing to be objective outside observer and complete our 'Following the RYCT approach checklist'.

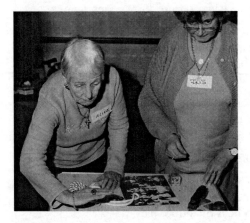 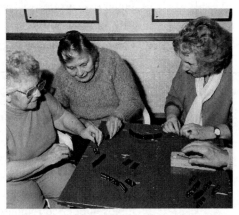

Figure 7.8: Alice turns out to be a skilful marbles player

Figure 7.9: A game of dominos in progress

SESSION 3: SCHOOLDAYS
Objectives

- To continue to develop the sense of belonging to the group.

- To introduce a new creative activity, improvisation.

- To re-experience some of the good and bad aspects of life at school.

- To build up a sense of common experience.

- To have some 'separate time' with the carers for discussion about how they are finding the project and for consciousness-raising.

This is the first session in which you might have some separate time for family carers. A way of using the 'teacher' to put the carers into a separate group is suggested below.

Outline plan
Triggers

- slates

- chalk

- school satchel

- school reports

- dipping pens

- a globe

- school tie and cap

- cane

- skipping rope

Opening

Welcome each family as they arrive and thank them for making the effort to come.

Show people to seats laid out in rows as in a classroom and tick a register as they arrive. Use props (e.g. blackboard) to suggest a schoolroom. A team member, probably one of the project workers, is in role as teacher, preferably quite fierce. It might be helpful here for the other project worker to be a link person, introducing the different activities and setting up the scenes with the teacher.

Teacher says 'Good morning children' and group replies 'Good morning Sir/Miss... Teacher takes the register, formally 'disciplining' anyone who is late, along lines recommended by the rest of the group!

Warm-up

Physical drill as done in school in the past – take suggestions from the group.

Pass a school satchel (or equivalent) round the group and invite each person to 'put something into it' which they might have taken to school and tell the group what it is (e.g. a penny, a sandwich, a pencil case, homework, cigarettes and a pin-up magazine(!), a geometry set, a catapult, a frog!).

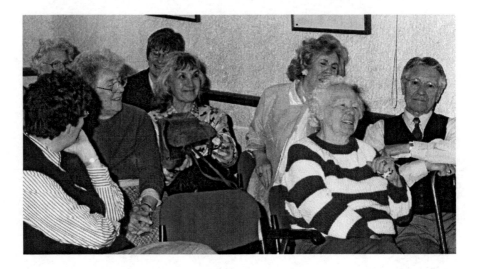

Figure 7.10: Group pass round a school satchel and remember something they took with them to school

Main activities

1. 'Teacher' comes out of role (or other project worker takes on the facilitator role) and asks: 'If this was a classroom when you were at school, what would be round the walls, what furniture would there be and how would it be arranged, what would the teacher wear, how would he or she deal with naughty or stupid children?' Group members call out short responses, which are picked up and reflected

back and developed by the 'teacher', who moves in and out of role as appropriate (or by the other project worker as facilitator) using other team members or participants as fellow actors.

2. 'Teacher', in role, gets everyone (who can) standing up and singing a well-known hymn, e.g. 'All things bright and beautiful', 'We plough the fields and scatter', or 'Onward Christian soldiers'. Ask group members if they have a favourite hymn or a poem they used to recite at school. Offer them the opportunity to do this.

3. Recall the times table and other measurements (chains, furlongs!). Recite all together. Once seven is seven, two sevens are fourteen, etc.

4. 'Teacher' moves in and out of role, asking the group to tell about any prizes they won, to come up to the front one at a time and receive them all over again in as formal a way as possible, with handshakes and rounds of applause for each one. Use this as an opportunity for people to remember past successes in school work, sports, reliability and regular attendance.

   Announce break time, and a chance to consider playground memories. 'Teacher' asks to see certain members of the group 'in my office' and calls out the names of the carers, as though they need a talking-to, and escorts them to another space.

Tea break: Provide tea and snack for both groups.

5a. In small groups, people with dementia and the team members and some volunteers play games connected with playtime at school using some of the objects from the previous session. They also explore any memorabilia members have brought from home (e.g. if anyone brings in a school report, you could read out extracts to the whole group). This helps everyone to visualise members of the group as youngsters.

5b. Meanwhile the group of family carers, meeting in a separate room, will be asked how they and the person they care for are finding the project. This is a chance to find out about any difficulties that participants are having, and to explain the RYCT ethos to family carers. If carers are tending to dominate and speak for the people they care for, the group leader can encourage carers to consider this issue and whether they can sometimes hold back. Suggest the idea of counting to five (or even ten!) before jumping in with all the answers, or use an exercise where the group of carers experience what it is like to be unable to find the words in time. (See outline plans for separate time with carers in Chapter 6.)

6. Bring the two groups together so carers can hear and see what their relative has been doing: playing games, sharing stories, etc.

Closing

Group leader gives a summary of what has been done.

Leader suggests an activity to do as 'homework' but not compulsory: make a drawing in their memory diaries of a teacher (loved or loathed), or a best school friend, or themselves as children.

Leader explains next week's theme: leaving school and starting work, and asks everyone to bring in one or two photographs or objects associated with their working lives, including apprenticeship papers, certificates, medals, etc.

Leader thanks everyone for being prepared to go back to school. Personal good-byes.

Session notes: Schooldays

Activities used today

- Chairs arranged in rows facing front, schoolroom style.

- Images of school placed on chairs.

- Teacher (Pam in role) took register, hymn standing (as possible), pass the satchel for a memory, X tables. Gave remembered prizes, discussed favourite school subjects.

- Looked at school photos, school reports and medals or prizes brought in.

- Heard a special story from Max about sporting medals.

- After tea, we split the group, with family carers meeting at different end of the room.

- Carers – explored RYCT ethos, reflections and feedback so far, gave ideas for reminiscence at home, given exercise: count to ten before speaking for partner.

- People with dementia and volunteers – drew favourite teachers or school environments.

- Sharing back in whole group, final song, reminder about next theme

Comments

- Small group gave more potential for hearing memories, we then shared these in whole group. James and Tom more settled.

- Good interaction between James, Max and Olive. They talked together for some time. The other James needs action and non-verbal methods of reminiscence, drawing not successful. Try something different next week.

- Very positive feedback for project from carers' group.

- All enjoyed being pupils – laughter and surprise.

- Good bringing in of photos and objects – well acknowledged by whole group.

Points to consider in future sessions

- Fred needs one-to-one attention for activities when he's away from Ena.

- Support good interaction between the people with dementia, which we observed today.

- Unable to check 'Following the RYCT approach checklist' – OT student absent.

- Diaries – need to remind/suggest use. Get feedback from group on this. Some difficulty in separating Tom, James and Fred – volunteers have important role here in engaging them in the activity provided.

SESSION 4: STARTING WORK AND WORKING LIVES

Objectives

- To appreciate past skills and achievements of members.

- To find shared memories and common ground between group members.

- To celebrate diversity and difference in members' experiences of work.

- To explore the humour in being young and inexperienced.

Outline plan

Triggers

- tools
- folding wooden ruler
- typewriter
- wage packet
- old money
- apprenticeship certificates
- aprons
- washing boards
- overalls

Opening

Greet each person as they arrive.

    Optional activity might be setting up imaginary or improvised 'clocking in' system.

Warm-up

Make a machine as a group and add noises associated with places of work. This is not as difficult as it sounds. One person starts making a simple repetitive action in the centre of the circle, perhaps adding a suitable clicking or thumping sound to go with it. Another person comes in and either copies what the first person is doing or adds a new sound or action. People gradually join in so that, together, they make a big noisy composite machine. N.B. It is important to make sure there is someone to support each of the people with dementia.

Main activities

1. Arrange seating in a circle to play 'What's my line?' Working in twos and threes, group members hear about one another's first jobs and prepare a mimed scene to show to the rest of the group, who try to guess what it was. This can be one very simple action, with all the

small group performing a single action together or taking different roles (e.g. apprentice and boss).

2. Working with the whole group, ask about the first pay packet. What did members spend their first pay on and how much was it? Make a note of the answers on a flip chart so you can see who was paid the least and most and relate it to the year when people started work.

Tea break: Prepare a sandwich with traditional filling wrapped in brown paper and an enamel mug of strong tea, or a traditional 'in-service' tea tray to take 'upstairs'!

3. Working in small groups, use the items that people have brought from home to elicit memories. Use these memories to produce a drawing, a chart or a piece of writing for the members with dementia that relates to their working lives (e.g. drawing a plan of the workplace, a picture of the person wearing what he or she wore to work, or of a workmate; a chart illustrating a process, or work roles or a story about the boss).

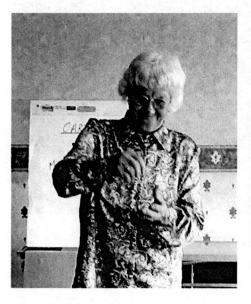

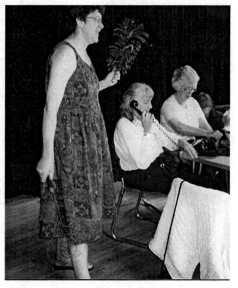

Figure 7.11: Maria in Bangor miming her work as a cook

Figure 7.12: Miming a scene set in a restaurant, with a part for everyone and props to help the show along

4. Have a selection of appropriate props and costumes available if possible such as overalls, headscarves, flat caps, hairnets, tools, spade or a typewriter, using your knowledge of the group members' previous occupations. Ask the members to work in three or four groups (focused around factories, offices, shops, catering, home, or whatever seems appropriate) and to prepare a short scene, tableau or a moving image about working life based on memories of one or more people in the group. Make sure everyone has a part, however small and encourage them to use the available props or improvise with whatever is to hand. Show each scene to the whole group and invite the observers to comment on what they see and recognise. Give a round of applause for each group and pick up particularly on the contributions made by the people with dementia.

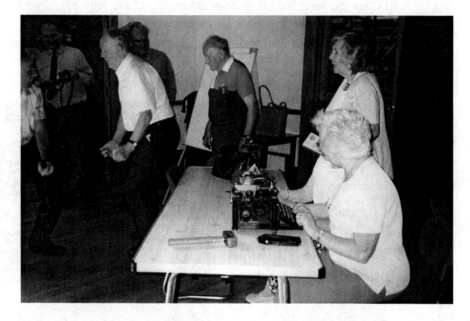

Figure 7.13: An improvised scene around memories of working in the docks

Closing

Leader reminds everyone about the highlights of the session, and asks participants to say what their favourite moment was.

Leader announces the next theme: going out, having fun, courting, cinema, and asks them to bring photos of themselves dressed up to go out, or for a favourite activity. Suggest they bring along if possible one or two objects associated with recreational activities from their youth.

Leader asks about dances people did when young and the music they danced to. Ask group members to bring in a cassette or CD of their favourite dance music.

Thanks people for coming and for being willing to join in the activities. Personal good-byes.

Session notes: Starting work and working lives

Activities used today

- Whole-group warm-up activity: 'busy' music on piano and actions reflecting work led by everyone in turn: owner of work memory, with rest of group following/copying.

- Created a group production line – really worked well with everyone participating.

- In small groups, shared apprenticeship certificates, etc. and memories of first jobs. Each group chose one job they'd discussed and mimed actions. Everyone else guessed the job.

- Tea tables set with artefacts to trigger work memories.

- People chose an object relating to a memory, shared memories at tables. Each group created an improvised scene set in a workplace: shop, office, factory, etc., and performed these for the rest of the group.

- Reminded everyone about break, Xmas party and next session theme.

Comments

- Actions to music developed well – everyone willing to take risks.

- Actions in circle developed into an inside circle of production line, then outer circle as factory walls. Live music created ideal rhythms.

- Work in small groups progressed well. Everyone enjoyed guessing mimed work, and majority were able to engage.

- We'd arranged the objects randomly, so a clear path to scenes of particular workplaces was not evident. Would have been much more productive if grouped thematically and people had chosen a theme relevant to their memory. The wide range of work experiences within groups also made strong representative scenes more difficult to produce.

- Three people with dementia were unable to engage fully with improvisation, but others responded very well, e.g. Iris, Max.

- Four of the carers seemed released through their play. Some tables continued to talk about the artefacts rather than create the environment through enactment.

Points to consider in future sessions

- Timing of break and use of role play with this group: is it likely to go better if tried in early part of afternoon?

SESSION 5: GOING OUT AND HAVING FUN
Objectives

- To recall past pleasures.

- To remember how it felt to be young, beautiful and fit.

- To share common experiences, such as cinema outings, first kiss, favourite dance halls, lipstick and perfumes.

- To celebrate idiosyncratic hobbies and interests.

- To key into the shared experience of the group.

If this is one of the sessions you have chosen for carers to have time on their own, arrange your programme so that there are good moments for them to withdraw and return to the group.

Outline plan
Triggers

- nylon stockings
- make-up
- shaving strop and razor
- jewellery
- gloves
- gramophone records
- theatre programmes
- scrap-books of film stars

Opening

Play some of the dance music mentioned by members as background music.

Welcome people with an invitation to dance and seat them in a circle around the room.

Have a display of clothes and accessories, perfumes, shaving gear, theatre programmes, fishing gear, walking boots, evening bags, etc. laid out in the centre of the circle. Invite group members to add what they have brought to this display.

Based on your knowledge of group members, prepare bags of objects for each group to explore, with a variety of textures and weights. Organise the groups around appropriate bags, for example, the men around a bag of fishing tackle, cycle parts, tools; women around a handbag with make-up, a silk scarf or a high-heeled dance shoe. Use this activity to move participants into different groupings.

Warm-up

Working in pairs, with one person 'mirroring' what his or her partner does, apply make-up, brush hair, shave, put on tie/necklace/ear-rings.

Some participants may be willing to 'model' the outfits they remember wearing to go out and their partner can explain what they are modelling.

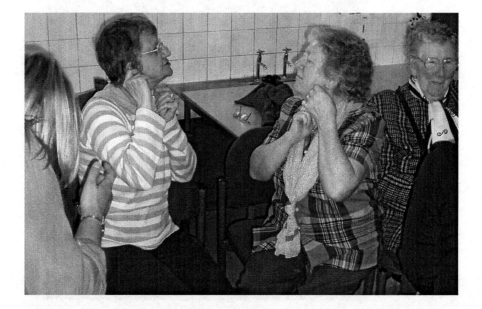

Figure 7.14: The mirroring exercise tried out in the Bradford group

Main activities

1. In small groups recall courting experiences, for example chat-up lines, monkey parade, flirting strategies, groups of girls eyeing the boys, wolf whistles, wallflowers, getting in late, parental advice to young people.

2. Alternatively, do this as a whole group, with girls on one side and boys on the other, making advances, advising one another on strategies and chat-up lines. It does not matter if numbers are uneven here, as everyone can call out their suggestions and comments, even if there are only two or three men in the group (as often seems to be the case) to carry out the advice!

3. Make any necessary furniture arrangements to make room for dancing. Using dance music suggested or brought by members, encourage team and group members who can to get up and dance. One option here is to have the men in each family get up and go across to invite their relative (or someone else!) to dance and to tell the group what they are remembering as they dance.

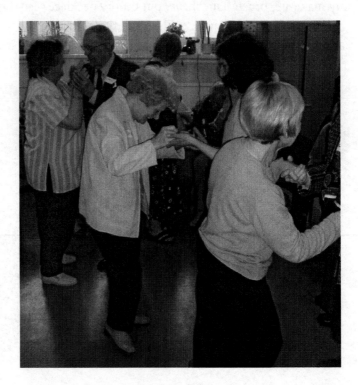

Figure 7.15: Mae checks her footwork while dancing

4. Rearrange the furniture in rows to represent cinema seating. Have
    everyone queue up to go in, pay at the desk and receive a ticket, show
    them to their seats torch in hand, cinema music playing. Ask people
    what film they have come to see – people call out favourite films.
    Facilitator calls out the type of film people are watching: 'It's a sad
    film', 'It's a funny film', 'It's a frightening film', 'It's a car chase' (you
    could make an appropriate sound track to facilitate this activity) and
    group members pretend to be the audience in each case, with
    appropriate facial expressions, body language, comments, etc.

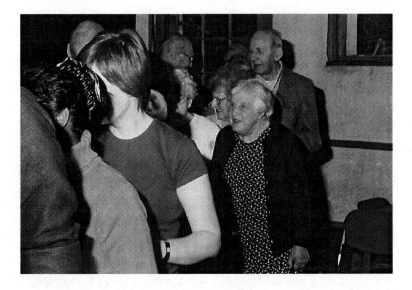

Figure 7.16: The whole group improvise a scene in a cinema queue

N.B. Memories of going to the cinema and favourite films and stars can
really warrant a session on its own and can certainly be pursued in the
reunion group.

Tea break: Serve ice creams if possible, peanuts, tea tray (apparently some
cinemas served you this in your seat!). Maybe share memories over tea of
kisses snatched in the cinema and sitting in the double seats for courting
couples.

Closing

Leader invites comments on memorable parts of the session. Leader announces next theme: weddings. Ask group members to bring in wedding photos, wedding menus, honeymoon bills, love letters, poems, etc. Be sensitive and work out how to involve anyone who has never married or same-sex couples.

Thank people for coming and for being willing to join in the activities. Personal good-byes.

Session notes: Going out and having fun

Activities used today

- Objects and clothes arranged on long table in middle of room to set the theme.

- Volunteers asked to find out from families their favourite dance music.

- Mirror work: pairs sat opposite each other and mimed getting ready for a night out.

- Men/women sat on different sides of the room. Men asked ladies for a dance. Dancing to piano, then 'Ladies' Excuse Me'.

- Memorable dance venues recalled, plus favourite bands and music.

- Tea and stories about meeting their partner for first time.

- Gave a choice between drawing their first meeting or role play.

- Presented small group plays and pictures to the rest of the group.

Comments

- Good atmosphere, no problems settling back after the Christmas break, people clearly feeling identified with the group.

- Moving into time in their lives when couples knew each other begins to reinforce the reason for doing reminiscence together even more strongly.

- Group at ease with each other, risks in revealing memories taking place.

- New discoveries for family members about each other, e.g. parents' weekend away together before marriage revealed to the two daughters in one family.

- Dancing and moving about a positive part of the session. Getting up and having a break from the concentration of listening is essential in this group.

- Role plays were impressive in that most had a go, all on-task for sharing memories about first meetings.

Points to consider in future sessions

- Carers split to happen at some stage, more for bonding than needing specific ideas on reminiscence.

- Couples seem content with ethos.

- Need to find out which couples have children for Session 7.

- Marlene (hospital staff OT) agreed to observe and complete 'Following the RYCT apprach checklist' from next session onwards.

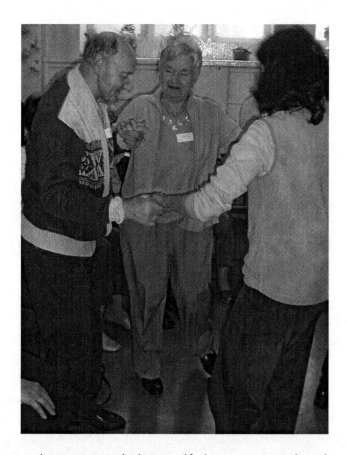

Figure 7.17 Audrey Lewis, group leader in Bradford, encourages a couple to take to the floor

SESSION 6: WEDDINGS
Objectives

- To remind caring spouses of the foundations of their relationship.

- To reinforce bonds with people alive or dead.

- To focus on the participants at a glamorous time in their lives.

- To share common experience.

Outline plan
Triggers

- marriage certificates

- wedding rings

- wedding photos

- sample wedding presents

- love letters

Opening

Welcome participants as though to a wedding, asking/telling them that they are relatives of the bride or groom, and showing them to the bride or groom's seats.

Have the seats set up in rows with an aisle in middle. Encourage them to act as guests, speculating about what the bride might be wearing, and how they feel about the forthcoming marriage.

Warm-up

All together facing front, mime getting ready for the wedding. Have a man and woman at front taking it in turn to do actions, with participants mirroring. Woman does hair, make-up, lipstick, skirt length, seams straight, etc. Man does shaving action, hair brushing, polishing shoes on trousers, fishing for wedding ring in his pocket. Both do buttonhole or bouquet adjustments.

Main activities

1. Two participants are asked to play 'bride and groom'. Give everyone else roles and ask them to take their places for the ceremony. Possible roles here are best man, vicar, bride's parents, jilted girl or boyfriend, drinking mate of groom or bridesmaid. Have bride and groom enter (to appropriate music, sung or played) and proceed up aisle and get married by someone in role of vicar/priest.

   Give group confetti or petals to throw, and words of advice for the couple if they feel like it. Everyone poses for a series of wedding photos and maybe speeches. Invite people to share wedding stories – pass a bride's head-dress to those with a wedding story to tell.

2. Working in small groups look at photos and objects brought from home. Choose one item for everyone to contribute to a 'Courting and Marriage' display. Make captions for these items.

3. Working as a whole group invite each person to add their contribution to the display. Leader makes encouraging comments about each item, bringing out links and celebrating difference. Take a photo of the display.

4. Make a note of the wedding date of each group member and arrange them in order on a flip chart with their names. Include the maiden names of the ladies.

   Tea break: Serve champagne and wedding cake, perhaps!

5. Using the displayed objects, make up a story about a wedding as a whole group, with everyone adding a sentence or just one word. For example, a team member might say 'And the bride was called...', then ask one of the people with dementia for a name, so they just say 'Mary' or 'Alice', but they are contributing.

6. In the whole group, make a wedding present list for an imaginary couple, each person adding something to the list. Alternatively, explore memories of wedding presents the group received, wedding traditions they observed, the trousseau they collected, honeymoon plans and, if people are willing, wedding night experiences!

Closing

Leader invites people to say what they will remember about the session.

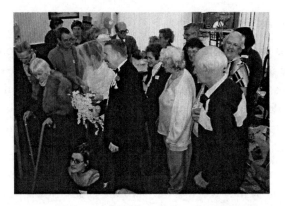

Figure 7.18: The wedding procession involves everyone in the group, and some have brought special clothes for the event

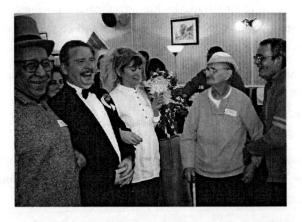

Figure 7.19: Re-enacting happy wedding memories reawakens strong positive emotions

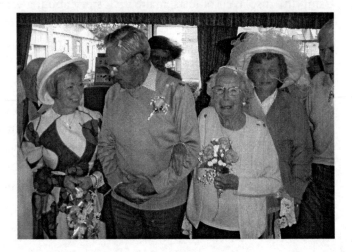

Figure 7.20: Posing for the family wedding photo in Bradford

Leader explains next week's theme: homes, gardens and animals, and asks everyone to bring in one or two objects associated with a memorable place where they have lived, photos or pictures of the place, the garden, animals they kept or anything else strongly associated with that place.

Thank people for coming and for sharing their memories. Personal good-byes.

Session Notes: Weddings

Activities used today

- Seated as families of bridegroom in church in two banks of pews, 'organ-type music' (tune: 'Sheep may safely graze') played by Olive and hummed by 'congregation'.

- Working in pairs, people checked their appearance (Hair OK? Seams straight? Lipstick not smudged? Tie nicely tied?)

- Asked people to volunteer for important roles (bride's parents, bridesmaids, etc.) and played out the ceremony, with break in the middle of service to allow everyone to give their advice to the 'happy couple'.

- Threw confetti and then posed for whole-group photos, everyone recalling a memory of a wedding, their own or someone else's.

- Tea.

- Shared photos, clothes, artefacts.

- Read out telegrams and cards people had brought in which they had kept.

- Placed bridal head-dress on each former bride and heard about her wedding.

- Recalled memorable gifts, honeymoons, unusual circumstances, etc.

- Songs performed at weddings were sung, some solos and some whole group.

- Reminded people about objects for next session and thanked for photos, wedding clothes, etc. brought in this week.

Comments

- Artefacts brought by nearly all and appreciated by others. There was much enjoyment in sharing and displaying these. Ceremony went well, group may have enjoyed more chance to comment in middle of service. Could have been stronger to re-marry some existing couple, but volunteer 'bridegroom' had come dressed so smartly in wedding clothes, so we went with that!

- During the photo call after wedding there was a nice sense of closeness and purpose in the throng. Being in role with a task that all could do provided a chance for a different way of relating in that space.

- They enjoyed taking roles and the improvised wedding speech was responded to well – no confusion evident.

- Theme had been well set from start of session, with repetitions to remind people with dementia what we were doing. Volunteers and carers at home with theme, and the resulting confidence enabled whole group to be part of the event.

Points to consider in future sessions
Need more observation and guidance for Fred to avoid another incident with Meg, who misconstrued his desire for contact with her and got upset. Problem defused within session. Allocate someone to be with him throughout session on one-to-one basis?

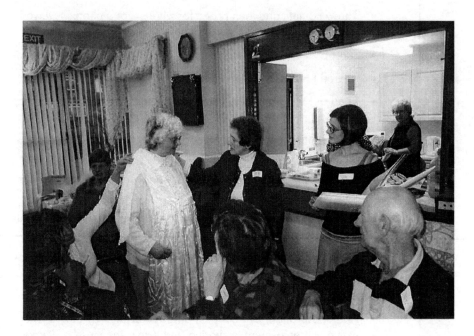

Figure 7.21: Holding up the original wedding dress to help trigger memories

SESSION 7: HOMES, GARDENS AND ANIMALS
Objectives

- To stimulate memories of the home environment in early married/adult life.

- To recall activities and skills associated with home life (DIY, gardening, decorating, sewing curtains, buying furniture, managing money and resources, looking after pets or knocking up shelves).

- To recapture the aspects of life at home.

If this is one of the sessions you have chosen for carers to have time on their own, arrange your programme so that there are good moments for them to withdraw and return to the group.

Outline plan

Triggers

- paintbrush and tins of paint

- garden tools

- rent books

- dog lead

- hammer and nails

- furniture catalogues

Opening

Welcome each family as they arrive. Thank them for coming. As you greet the people, mention something you already know about them related to places they have lived.

Show people to seats at small tables, seating people in appropriate groups based on your experience from previous sessions, each group with a member of the project team.

Warm-up

In turn, people mime actions, such as washing, digging, washing up, mopping, painting walls, polishing, stroking the cat, patting the dog or 'winding' the baby. The rest of the group copy the actions.

If this is one of the sessions you have chosen where carers are having separate time, the facilitator can announce that he or she needs their help at this point, and take the carers into another room. If you are having a 'show', they will need to return in time to be in 'the audience' (see below, number 4).

Main activities

1. Working in small groups, look at what people have brought in. Encourage memories of places, surroundings, gardens, homes and explore details. For example discuss living with parents, first independent homes, prefabs and other temporary post-war homes, work-related homes, service homes and barracks, ships, caravans.

    If there is an outdoor space to work in, this is a good session to go there and offer some outdoor activities, such as digging, planting, shelling peas, hulling strawberries or whatever is in season, or hanging out the washing.

    Sharing with whole group: each group to feed back a taste of what they did.

2. Home chores, activities and projects. Working in small groups use triggers such as old magazines, books and advertisements to elicit memories of the things people did to – and in – their homes and gardens, such as buying furniture, hire purchase; making ends meet; decorating, home improvements; making clothes for the children; things grown in the garden; animals kept, rabbits, pigeons, poultry, pigs, pets, and animals removed, spiders, mice, rats, foxes).

3. Sharing with the whole group: each group mime one of the activities they have remembered for others in the group to guess.

    Tea break: If possible use some traditional china (which might have been given as a wedding present) or enamel mugs (as used in the shed) or picnic cups (as taken to the allotment).

4. An animal show. Working in small groups, find out about the place of animals in members' lives. Encourage each person to choose an animal to bring to an imaginary show. Celebrate memories of animals by

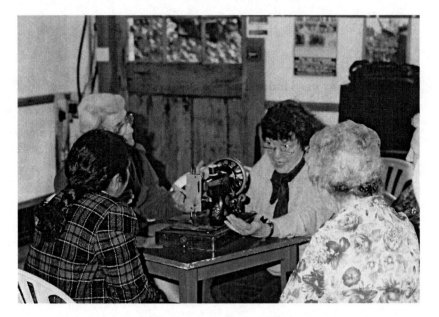

Figure 7.22: The sewing machine evokes memories of making clothes for children, making curtains and covers and, for some people, work before marriage as seamstresses

bringing them into a 'show ring'; each person says something about the animal and why they have brought them. (This can include pets, farm animals, animals hunted, imaginary pets, or even pests like mice or foxes that they have brought to the show to get rid of.)

5. Song session. In the whole group, think about any songs about animals and sing them. This can be done in two groups as a competition to see which group can think of the most!

Closing

Leader invites younger people in the room to comment on what they have learned from older people's memories.

Leader announces next week's theme: 'The next generation', and asks people to bring in pictures of their children, nieces, nephews or other babies, children they have looked after, known or loved.

Thanks. Personal good-byes.

Session notes: Homes, gardens and animals

Activities used today

- Seats arranged in a circle with artefacts on table across centre.

- Introduced the theme and asked everyone to choose an object with an associated memory to share in whole group.

- Group warm-up: actions associated with first homes – polishing floor, cleaning windows, sewing curtains, painting walls, etc., played as follow-my-leader, taking turns in leading.

- Geographical exercise – went N, S, E, W, to location of first homes. People asked for addresses and some people remembered phone numbers too!

- Common first home experiences shared: living with parents, flat, prefab, home with garden, etc.

- Tea in groups arranged on basis of similar experiences.

- After tea, we split the group.

- Carers looked at ideas for joint activities to do at home to reinforce positive interactions with a purpose, e.g. *Radio Times* – choose a TV or radio programme together. Carers are a strong group with good skills, worthwhile to give them opportunity to bond, share experiences, and share input on possible positive joint activities at home.

- People with dementia did drawings with volunteers relating to memories of gardens and homes.

Comments

- Actions of household tasks: we needed to elicit more information before doing the actions and moving around in space. Perhaps we could have started the actions sitting down to clarify structure of the exercise, and then started moving in the space, requesting further suggestions for actions from the group.

- Focus for the session difficult to keep, either because memories around first homes were not so clear, or maybe because we as leaders were not clear enough in guidance, i.e. did we want to explore the idea of different roles in the household or alternatively to be shown the specific tasks people did?

- Exercise could have developed more strongly if we'd been better prepared and coordinated.

- Group were interested in each other's experiences and contrasted mother-in-law memories, family relationships, places lived. Most work well when up and moving – geographical exercise went well, actions on the floor entered into enthusiastically.

- Carers were at ease with splitting the group, and good bonding taking place.
- Individuals had opportunity to talk with leader one-to-one.
- Important information shared in this setting re dyslexia and also isolation experienced.
- People with dementia kept concentration for a short period, but three required one-to-one attention during this time.
- Activity of drawing was a good way of recapitulating memories shared today for some.
- Participation varied. Max said that he was enjoying the development of a special relationship with a volunteer, through powerful early memories being shared.

Points to consider in future sessions

- Whole-group work was particularly effective today because there were some absentees. The slightly smaller/closer circle helped communication.
- We need to discuss one-to-one work, especially briefing volunteers on what to do when group divides to allow time for separate carers' group.

SESSION 8: THE NEXT GENERATION – BABIES AND CHILDREN
Objectives

- To recall memories of looking after babies and children, and memories associated with them, such as love, playfulness, being big and strong compared to them, the smell and feel of babies, noise and movement, tickling, chasing, hide and seek, kissing it better and naughtiness.
- To express opinions about something that affects everyone (we have all been cared for as babies and children, and most of us have cared for them too).
- To revisit past competence and responsibilities, and maybe remind spouses and sons and daughters who are now carers how things used to be very different.

If this is one of the sessions you have chosen for carers to have time on their own, arrange your programme so that there are good moments for them to withdraw and return to the group.

Outline plan

Triggers

- old-fashioned feeding bottle
- nappy
- big safety pin
- bibs
- rattles
- teddies
- rose-hip oil
- weighing book
- national dried milk
- welfare orange juice bottle
- baby name book
- Christening gown
- matinee jacket
- knitting patterns
- photos of babies in old-fashioned baby clothes

Opening

Greet people as they arrive and show them 'the new baby' (doll) in a cot or pram or cradle or in volunteer's arms (a real one might be even better!). Everyone is invited to choose a name and sex for the baby as they come in.

Leader invites each person in turn to share the name they'd give the baby and the gift they would give it as a fairy godmother (e.g. lots of love, money, a rabbit, cuddles, a locket, £1000, etc.).

Warm-up

Mime and copy actions relating to babies (e.g. patting and winding the baby, rocking the baby, giving medicine, encouraging the toddler to walk).

Main activities

1. Working in small groups, ask people to choose an object from the display, and talk about memories associated with the item in their group. Share stories with the whole group.

2. Remember the sayings (e.g. spare the rod and spoil the child) and the dos and don'ts of child rearing (e.g. not picking up, feeding on the hour, old wives' tales, home remedies, gripe water, what to feed babies, etc.) in the whole group. Changing attitudes (Dr Spock, etc.) and being a grandparent. Leader asks older people in the group for their opinions about childrearing today. Make a record of their advice to new parents today.

Tea break: Serve rusks and Ribena perhaps?! Use the tea-break to remember all the clever ways they got their babies to eat, such as 'Down the red lane!' or 'Here comes the train into the tunnel'.

3. Return to small groups to 'bath the baby'. Have enough bowls, dolls and towels for each family to have a go, clothes to put on the babies after they are bathed. Alternatively, have one bath and one doll and let people have a turn at showing their skill and methods. Encourage people to talk about memories of bathing babies, or being bathed as small children.

4. What has happened to the babies and children participants looked after? In small groups, each person tell about one baby or child they cared about and say what happened to them when they grew up. Share these stories with the whole group. (This is a chance for people who have been parents to talk with pride about their grown-up children; project team need to make sure that those without children of their own feel included, so it is important to open up the topic to cover nieces and nephews and the children of close friends.)

5. Working as a whole group, remember songs sung to babies and favourite stories told to children. Invite people to sing the songs they remember to everyone, or tell the stories.

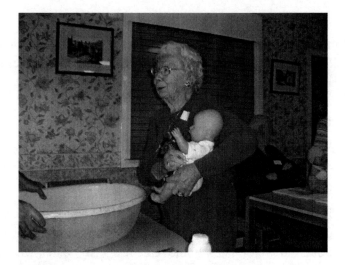

Figure 7.23: Bathing the baby remembered in the Bradford group

Closing

Leader facilitates summing up, asking group for their moments to remember from the session.

Leader announces next week's theme: 'Food and cooking', and discusses suggestions about what food the group would like to make, and eat, next week.

Ask people to bring aprons and table decorations (candles, flowers, fancy plates, doilies, napkins and rings) or drinks for next week.

Thanks and personal good-byes.

Session notes: The next generation – babies and children

Activities used today

- Welcome and recap on previous sessions: a useful summary and confirmation of our work together to date.

- Artefacts relating to babies and their upbringing, pram and dolls were placed around the room.

- Asked people to recall songs sung as/to children, lullabies, etc.

- Did actions to music relating to dandling, burping, rocking, soothing babies.

- Went around circle hearing names their babies were called, reasons for choice of name and meanings of these names.

- Discussed different ways of raising babies, with Asian/Eastern binding and massage input from Trinidad and India. All this took a long time, but people were absolutely held by it.

- Everyone chose an artefact that had a meaning for them and took that into small groups for tea and sharing memories.

- We bathed the dolls (real water used) while recalling bath times and rituals with their own babies.

- Fed back briefly to whole group the essence of the stories shared in small groups.

- Told them theme for the next session and asked them to bring favourite recipe books, etc.

Comments

- Spent some time around the circle to include all who wished to contribute, losing a little of the pace but still engaging memories shared.

- In the post-session discussion we decided to try other methods of whole-group discussion – in particular using one input to trigger another, rather than taking turns around the whole circle.

- Laughs and engagement from unexpected sources for doll washing – sensory stimulus of water and soap essential and need more activities for people with severe dementia.

- Would have been good to have some words for songs written down as the more interesting songs were only sung by one or two people.

- Very relaxed opening to session, informal sharing. People enjoyed listening to each other on the baby names they had chosen – it is a very personal thing and hearing the reasons for choosing names contributed to building trust in the group.

Points to consider in future sessions

- Session was late to start as one leader was held up. Would have been better to start without her.

- The informal opening worked well, but left limited time to do other things.

- Fred was shadowed by a volunteer who worked with him on a one-to-one basis to monitor behaviour to others in the group. We need to ensure that this task is shared.

SESSION 9: FOOD AND COOKING
Objectives

- To recall the good feelings associated with food and eating.

- To make use of taste, textures and smell as memory triggers.

- To provide an opportunity to recall and practise old skills.

- To co-operate with others in a practical task.

Outline plan

Triggers

- recipe books

- wooden spoons and mixing bowls

- tea trays laid out with crockery

- cake stand

Opening

Greet people as they come in, reminding them of the plan to prepare some food this week.

Take them to seats at tables where ingredients and utensils are laid out for preparing something to cook, preferably with two or three options, such as scones, bread, fairy cakes.

Explain to whole group what they will be cooking and eating, giving choices based on preferences where possible. Suggest that everyone puts on aprons – have some spares in case people have forgotten to bring them.

Main activities

1. In small groups, make something which can be ready within the group period, and can be served to the group (small sponge cakes, bread, scones) or uncooked food like fruit salad or sandwiches. Make sure the people with dementia (including the men) are given as much responsibility as possible and can make a meaningful contribution.

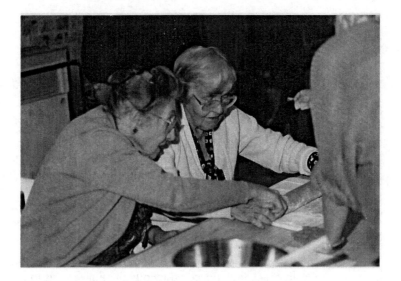

Figure 7.24: Sybil and Betty, her friend, make pastry in the group

2. Arrange a table attractively, using whatever people have brought.
    Include flowers and candles, depending on the season. Make the
    arranging of the table and bringing food to it a part of the activity,
    with everyone who can doing their bit. Maybe have music playing
    while this activity goes on.

3. Gather as a whole group (while food is cooking or afterwards) and
    pass a plate or bowl around. Invite everyone in turn to put in an
    imaginary favourite (or least favourite) food, perhaps one cooked by
    Mum or Gran, or their own 'specials'. Each person says why they
    have chosen that food.

4. Invite people to sit round the table and share what has been prepared
    and whatever drinks have been brought in. Create a party atmosphere,
    with speeches and songs. Find something to celebrate for everyone,
    e.g. anniversary, birthday last/next month, feeling better after illness,
    having a grandchild, having a holiday, being here.

Closing

Final 'speech' to say good-bye to everyone and thank them for coming to the
party.

Invite people to bring along objects and pictures next time connected
with holidays and journeys.

Session notes: Food and cooking

Activities used today

- Set up in advance: flip chart and pens; tables for food preparation; utensils to do with cooking; semi-prepared ingredients for making pancakes and fairy cakes; some prepared bread dough for people to knead.

- Split group to give carers a separate session for first half, focusing on their skills as carers, and encouraging them to prepare something at home with the person with dementia to bring back to the group. Asked the carers to explore how they are reacting to what their relative does at home, including how they respond to efforts at washing up, drying, table laying, etc.

- This was a consciousness-raising session in which the main idea was to check if carers could try out alternative ways to keep their relatives feeling good about themselves and not put down. Lots of new resolutions were made and some people said they had already been implementing the 'counting to ten before speaking' strategy with some success.

- Parallel group: began by eliciting ideas from group of people with dementia about ingredients needed for each recipe and then recorded their remembered methods on flip chart.

- Arranged people in groups with volunteers to help each group. Each table made one of the recipes, everyone taking turns to do things like blend the ingredients, mixing, chopping, measuring out, etc. While they did this, people shared memories of preparing food in the past or watching their mothers and what they did as children.

- While food was cooking we passed round 'smell bags 'and people guessed what was inside. People with dementia and volunteers prepared the table and decorated it really nicely.

- Break, with some of the cooked food to share. The whole group came together and sat around the long table.

- While pancakes were being cooked, the cooking group fed back to carers what they had been doing. We finished with 'pass the plate' exercise where everyone shared what their favourite food was, when they were young or now.

Comments

- This session worked well and allowed the people with dementia to relate more to each other and work as a team.

- The men got on particularly well, with good volunteer support.

- People were well able to remember past skills and some said they would like to do more at home as a result, especially Iris.

- It was good to be able to feed back to carers and for them to see the results of their people's efforts and to celebrate this together.

Points to consider for future sessions

- We need to note that the men had a very positive response to today's activity and look for ways to help them relate well to one another like this in other sessions. This might help them keep contact when project is finished and between reunion group meetings.

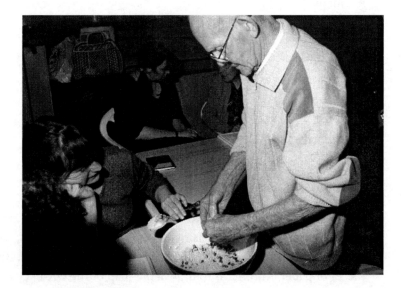

Figure 7.25: George bakes with Caroline's help

SESSION 10: HOLIDAYS AND TRAVEL
Objectives

- To remind people of the richness of their lives and their own past competence and sense of adventure.

- To share enthusiasms and favourite places and to remember the pleasures and disasters of holidays and journeys.

- To validate the life experience of people who have come from other countries.

If this is one of the sessions you have chosen for carers to have time on their own, arrange your programme so that there are good moments for them to withdraw and return to the group.

Outline plan

Triggers

- souvenirs
- leather suitcase
- rucksack
- maps
- bicycle parts
- stick of rock
- shells
- postcards
- swimsuits

Opening

Find a way to indicate that the room is a map of the UK – or perhaps the world. One way to do this is using labels saying North, South, East and West, or putting places such as John O'Groats, Land's End, London, Belfast, etc. on pieces of paper. Another is to draw a big map of the UK in chalk around the whole floor.

As people come in, greet them warmly, then explain that the room is a map and invite them to choose a place on the 'map' – outside the UK if they like – connected with a holiday memory or a place they have travelled to or lived. Take chairs to the places people have chosen.

Warm-up

In a circle as a whole group, follow the leader (or passing on the lead if appropriate) with actions for swimming, paddling, waving, towelling, digging, stone skimming, diving, eating fish and chips, bat and ball games, golf.

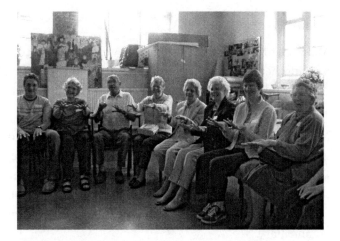

Figure 7.26: Warm-up exercises in the Bradford group: making waves

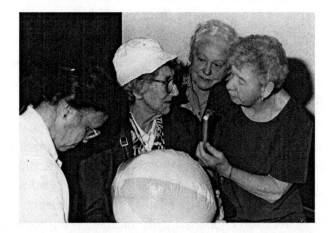

Figure 7.27: Edith and volunteers bring seaside memories to life

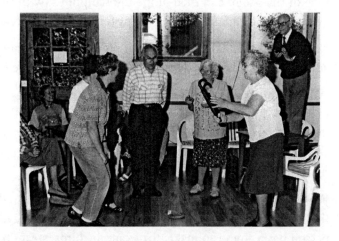

Figure 7.28: Taking a photo on the beach: an improvisation in the London group

Main activities

1. Make small groups from the people who have chosen places near to one another, and get them to say something about the place they have chosen and why. See if there are common memories of holidays and special places.

2. Members of the project team work with each small group to create a 'still photograph' based on one of the stories that have come up. People in the group pose as people in the memory; items from the display can be used as props. Each small group presents their still photo to the whole group, with an explanatory caption or commentary.

3. A member of the project team takes a real photo of each group's enactment of a photo and these should be processed so they can be shown at the next session.

4. Working with the whole group, pass round a basket or hamper and ask everyone to put in an item of food or drink that they might take on a holiday picnic or when travelling.

5. Bring in a bag of sand and some large pieces of plastic to cover the tables, also jugs for water and small buckets or cups. If possible, also bring seashells, little flags and fir cones for decoration. Work in small groups to prepare sand sculptures, collages or castles. This is an opportunity for creativity related to past experience. People may want to model a fort connected with wartime experience or a place they travelled to as adults (one couple built a pyramid on the River Nile!) One of the group can then judge the sculptures (with small prizes for everyone) and then invite all groups for tea and ice-cream.

Tea break: Serve ice-cream if possible, or picnic tea (with hamper?). Or serve exotic snacks from countries where people have either lived or holidayed.

6. Working in small groups, help everyone to make a postcard from a place they have been remembering. People can draw the picture on the card, decide who it is going to be sent to, add a message, the address, the date they are remembering or today's date, and draw a remembered or imaginary stamp.

7. Working with the whole group make a 'sound collage' that relates to the stories people have told about holidays and/or travelling. Each person has a sound to make, for example, birds, steam train, bus

conductors, crickets, sea, brass band, streams, steamers, hooters, sellers, rain and thunder. The leader acts as conductor, bringing in the different groups at different times, and indicating loud and soft, fast and slow.

8. Recall songs associated with holidays and travel and sing together. Maybe arrange chairs in pairs as though in a charabanc, or in eights with four facing opposite four as if in a train compartment, for this activity to evoke memories of the return journey.

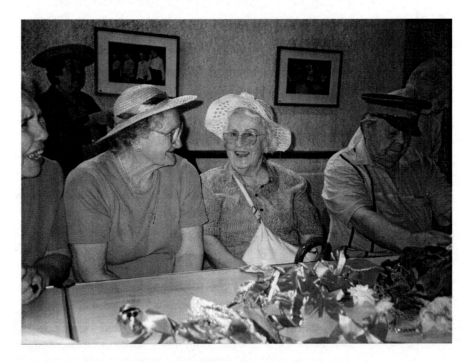

Figure 7.29: Suitable hats for a seaside trip with a coach driver

Closing

Leader facilitates summing up and invites people to read out their postcard messages to the group.

Remind the family carers that next week they should prepare and bring their appreciation of their person or the summary of their shared life and the good times they have had together. Remind them to bring in a few mementos (photos, documents, letters or objects) to help with the story.

Thanks and personal good-byes.

Session notes: Holidays and travel

Activities used today

- Warm-up with holiday actions and music, everyone taking it in turn to lead.

- People went North, South, East, West to holiday destinations and talked in small groups where they ended up, sharing experiences and holiday memories.

- Fed back to large group with songs people remembered.

- Tea and writing postcards from the holiday destination.

- Scenes in picture postcards formed into scenes and role plays.

- Mentioned we are nearly at the end of the programme.

- Reminded carers to prepare celebrations of the person they come with for next week.

Comments

- NSEW gave new combinations of people mixing and very positive interactions resulting.

- More than usual involvement in the warm-up of holiday actions shown by the people with dementia.

- A very happy atmosphere generated by the group during the session, in response to theme, activities and their engagement with each other.

- The final section, where everyone improvised their memories, went slightly anarchic, but it was all received with great humour.

- Some tension present due to aggressive body language and sometimes words of Fred. Team today worked well in preventing close proximity of concerned individuals, way-laying build up of conflict.

- Less up-front participants were relaxed and open today, participating from their chairs or moving across the room for the NSEW exercise. Much action and animation in the room. Down on volunteers today, but those who were there were well able to support reminiscing and comprehension.

- No expressions of concern about end of programme voiced. The reunion group is soon after the final session, and this is probably reassuring them that they can carry on with reminiscence activities and on-going relationships with group members.

Points to consider in future sessions

- Possibly workers or volunteers could do an appreciation of how they have come to know and appreciate the participants with dementia to be read out during last sessions. Workers to consider this for possible trial next week.

- Not all the 'Hopes and fears' were collected in Session 1: we need to make sure we do this, so everyone can look at what they said when we come to Session 12.

- This afternoon the group enjoyed a slow and social start to activities, although workers felt we needed to begin activity on time. People at ease with a social informal start – need to think carefully about pace and timing.

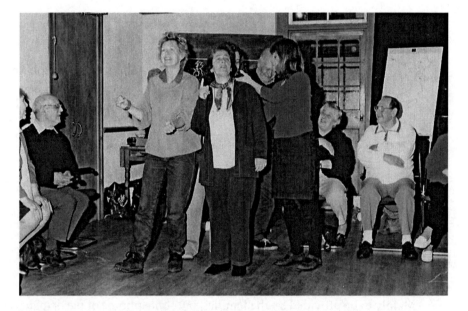

Figure 7.30: Improvising a family holiday journey remembered by one of the group

SESSION 11: CELEBRATION
Objectives

- To give the carers the opportunity to draw together what has been explored throughout the project concerning their person's life and character and to offer the same opportunity to the people with dementia.

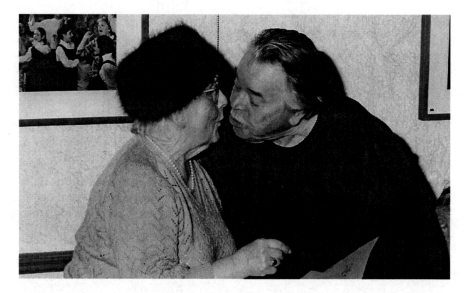

Figure 7.31: Inge is touched by the Valentine card Bill has made for her in the group

- To encourage the carers to think positively about their person and to affirm their relationship.

- To encourage the carers to put the present situation in a longer-term context of the life of the person with dementia and their relationship over time.

- To offer possibilities for carers, together with their person with dementia, to prepare something for the group.

Outline plan

Triggers

Mainly to be provided by the families, but some photos of participants taken during the project will be helpful. (See note under main activity 4 about showing a film/video record of edited highlights of the project to help remind participants what the group has done before they take their evaluation forms to fill in.)

Opening

As people arrive, greet them warmly and show the photos taken in the previous session (recording the 'still photographs' each group made based on memories of holidays and travel). Check if the carers have prepared something to share. If they have not, perhaps take a few moments to talk through with them some of the stories and experiences of their person which have emerged over the weeks. Use their project record book to help here if they have completed one. Alternatively, offer them the option of preparing something for the next and final session instead.

Main activities

1. Invite the families in turn to present what they have prepared: showing the objects, documents or photos they have brought in and an appreciation of their person.

2. As each person is appreciated, the group members can add what they have liked about that person and some of the stories they have shared or activities they have done together. It would be good to have a song connected with each person from one of the topics explored during the project.

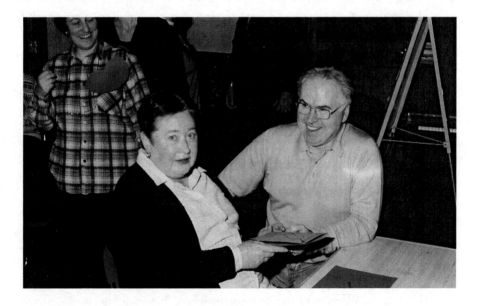

Figure 7.32: Valentine cards are made by participants and carers to express their love and affection

Tea break: Remind people of what they said was their favourite childhood dish in the cooking session.

3. 'Lifelines': in the second half of the session, each family, helped by volunteers and project workers, can prepare a lifeline of the person with dementia, showing major events and important turning points and achievements. This can be done in a variety of ways, but the simplest is to draw a line and divide it into eight or ten sections, roughly representing decades or life stages. Then start writing important things that happened into each section or doing small drawings above and below the line.

4. If you have made a film of the sessions or photographed the activities, it is a good idea to have this material available in this session. It will help families to remember what the project has covered and to complete the questionnaire (see below). Alternatively, such a film record can be shown in the final session as a means of rounding off the project.

Closing

Give out evaluation forms and ask people to complete them at home and bring them to the next and final session. It is a good idea to give each family two forms, so that the people with dementia have their own form to complete, though they may need some help with this from their carer or a volunteer or friend. (You will find the evaluation form in the Appendix.)

See Adaptions for 'Reminiscence Alone' Groups section later in this chapter for an alternative Session 11 without family carers.

Session notes: Celebration

Activities used today

- Physical warm-up – cold weather, snow balls, lots of activity. Everyone massaged each other's backs in a circle (then turning round and massaging person standing on other side) and enjoyed it!

- In small groups chose and talked about objects from the Keeping Warm in Winter Reminiscence Box. Shared these memories in the big circle.

- Tea and cakes served.

- Last part of session was listening to 'celebrations' – cherished memories of good times together from carers.

- Gave out evaluation forms and asked families to complete these and bring them to the final session.

Comments

- Very good atmosphere, relaxed and enjoyable. Much laughter at Lil being the snowman who melted! Lots of talk about warming foods, Aga ovens, etc. with plenty of cross-group discussion.

- Very pleased that so many carers had taken the task seriously and written or told such wonderful appreciations of their loved ones. This worked especially well where carers had prepared something in writing to read out. This seemed to give even more impact to what they said and the people with dementia concerned lit up. One highlight was a piece John and Iris had prepared together about the pleasure they had had on their caravan holidays and their sense of freedom when they set off. That sparked James's family to talk about their caravan and camping holidays together and they played out for us (with James as driver) one hilarious memory of a seaside near-disaster. Simon talked about what a lot he had learned from Nell and how important she was for him.

Points to consider for future sessions

- It might be good to model the 'appreciation of your person' idea over two sessions.

- Had the impression that some people had not quite grasped it and so had not prepared. If they had seen it done in the previous session, they might have been able to produce something even more positive than spontaneous offerings.

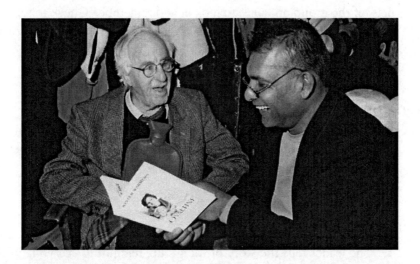

Figure 7.33: Colin enjoys a remembered story about keeping warm in winter read by Adrian Dassrath, community psychiatric nurse linked with the RYCT London project

SESSION 12: ROUNDING UP AND EVALUATION
Objectives

- To hear from the group about what the sessions have meant to them.

- To reminisce as a group about what they have done together over the weeks.

- To affirm the group and its achievements.

- To confirm arrangements about a reunion.

Outline plan

Triggers

- photos of the project

- written work and drawings by participants

- a display of the families' record books of the project

- film/video record of the project

Opening

Welcome people, and direct them to small groups. Have photos and 'products' of the group on tables to look at and remember. Check to see if people have filled in and brought back the evaluation form. If not, produce another copy and help them to do so.

Warm-up

In a circle, and all at the same time, invite people to say something to the people sitting on both sides of them about how they will remember them or about how their presence in the group has made a difference.

Main activities

1. The leader tells the story of the group, reminding everyone of the things they have done. The photos of previous sessions are shown, and passed round – if you have used video, watch some extracts if you did not show it in the previous session. Participants are invited to comment.

2. The leader asks people to share in small groups what they have put on the evaluation form, and asks for feedback to the whole group in the form of a summary from one person in each group. The leader should make it clear that people are entitled to say what they did not like as well as what they did, and that negative responses can be positive for the project as a whole, in that they can help the team do better next time. The leader should thank all the respondents for their comments.

3. An optional activity is for the whole group to make a series of tableaux, or still images representing the sessions one by one. For example the leader calls out 'the workdays session' and everyone poses in a still position connected to that theme. Leave time for people to look at what others are doing by dividing the group in two and letting half look at the other half's tableau and then swapping over.

4. Leader presents everyone with an individual certificate of participation, which is formally presented and applauded.

Tea party: Mark the ending of the group with a special tea and cakes. Allow time for songs and speeches. Participants can be given opportunities to perform, repeating things they have done in earlier sessions.

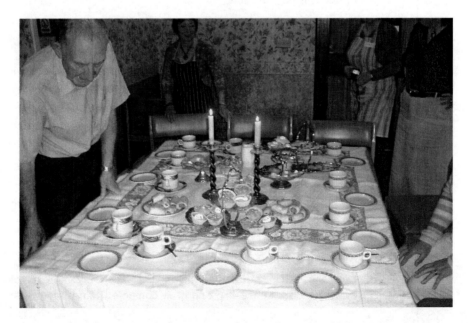

Figure 7.34: Putting the finishing touches to a festive tea party in the Bradford group

Closing

How many ways can the group think of to say good-bye?

Follow the leader initially, but allow participants to think of a new one and everyone does that until a new idea surfaces.

Leader gives formal thanks to everyone, for making the effort to come, for participating in the activities, and for sharing their stories.

Leader announces the reunion group, or plans for one, where applicable, giving out written information concerning dates, times and venues if available. Otherwise, an invitation can be offered to an event or meeting on a given future date, so that participants can definitely see one another again.

Personal warm good-bye to each person as they leave.

Session notes: Rounding up and evaluation

Activities used today

- Welcome into circle.
- Sum up of the content of all the sessions with personal references to group members' contributions and specific photos/items brought for the group.
- Asked people to share something memorable about the project – first in pairs and then feeding back into whole group.
- Video excerpts shown of different weeks of the project, and photos of sessions passed round.
- Tea.
- The group split after tea.
- Carers read out extracts from their evaluation forms and gave feedback on their reactions to the project and hopes for the future.
- The people with dementia sang favourite songs around the piano, one song for each of the themes explored during the project, and shared additional memories of the project.
- Whole group came together to share feedback.
- Reminded everyone about the monthly reunion club.
- Good-bye songs as a whole group.
- Farewells and thanks.

Comments

- Everyone liked the photos. Video good but screen very small, so not everyone able to see it properly. A contented atmosphere with people talking of the pleasure taken in activities, in laughter, and in seeing your person in a different light.

- The people with dementia responded well to songs covering the sequence of themes. This had the power to remind people of all the themes we had covered, which then led to improvised actions that we had used during the sessions (e.g. work mimes, washing the baby) and also additional verbal reminiscences. Music has been one of the most stimulating ways to share memories and group interactions. There were no signs of stress when the group split. Maybe singing together around the piano was helpful – it seemed a comfortable and comforting activity.

- Evaluations from carers were positive. Pat particularly amazed by how her husband came out of himself and appreciating how we helped him to participate.

- Most people said they would take up the offer to join the monthly reminiscence reunion club.

- Debrief with staff and volunteers was very powerful. People terrifically positive and upbeat about the project and what they think it is doing for participants. Good preparation, including the home visits, very worthwhile, and that the input for carers had been crucial.

Points to consider in future

- The role of volunteers is very important for participants needing one-to-one interaction to maximise what they can achieve.

- The role of multi-sensory stimulation is crucial when people are more severely impaired. We need to use the visual, the aural, oral, tactile and the kinaesthetic – to maximise the potential participation for the people with dementia.

- The role of music strengthens, as does dancing, as a shared activity.

- We had a very positive group dynamic, but we felt that at least two extra sessions would have enabled stronger consolidation of understanding and taking on the idea of reminiscence.

ADAPTATIONS FOR 'REMINISCENCE ALONE' GROUPS

You will find that you can use the same timetable of 12 sessions with people with dementia who come to the sessions without a family carer. The same guidelines apply, as do the RYCT essentials outlined at the beginning of the manual. The same themes and activities work well in these groups, but there are some differences when working with people with dementia 'alone' and we have suggested an alternative Session 11 (below) which can be run without family carers.

Bringing objects from home

Both because participants tend to be forgetful, and because family carers who are not coming to meetings do not always understand what is required, the team have to find ways to organise the bringing of objects from home. They also need to look after what is brought and make sure that it is taken home safely. One group produced a weekly letter for participants to take home, letting families know the theme for the next session and suggesting suitable objects, photos, certificates, etc. that could be brought in. Where carers came to collect participants, the letter was handed over in person, with some explanation and encouragement.

Not all participants will have family members taking an active interest in the project, and the team can help by finding objects or images (these can be from the Internet) likely to trigger memories for individuals. For example, a facilitator brought in a map for someone who came from Italy. This person could not recall the name of the place she came from, but she could recognise the name when she saw it on the map.

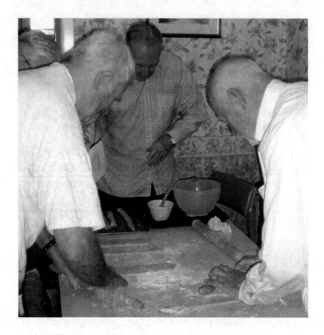

Figure 7.35: The men in the Bradford 'Reminiscence Alone' group making sausage rolls

Mime and improvisation

We have learned from experience that mime and improvisation work as well, if not better, in Reminiscence Alone groups than in joint groups. People with dementia often enjoy mime and improvisation or may enjoy directing volunteers to act out their story. In one group there was a woman who had worked as an escort on buses taking children with special needs to school. She directed other people to play the roles of the driver and children on the bus, while she herself played the escort, and the resulting improvisation was great fun for everyone. This reminded another participant of being an ambulance driver in the war and this led to a further improvisation. Volunteers with similar background or experience can be a great resource. For example a participant with dementia who had worked in a hospital was paired with a volunteer who had a hospital background and together they were able to produce a very good mime of taking blood pressure. This is an example of the body remembering the actions and reproducing them accurately.

Anxiety

Some people with dementia are more likely to feel anxious when attending a group alone, and when anxiety levels rise, they cannot concentrate on the activities unless they are reassured. Members of the project team need to be quick to spot anxiety, and to learn how to provide effective reassurance. One-to-one attention is nearly always essential, and the team need to discuss and share the different approaches that they are using to reassure anxious participants.

Participating and taking the lead

Some people with dementia seem to feel freer to participate and take the lead when they are apart from their family carers. The group can be a rare opportunity to revisit the experience of being in charge, something that tends to be lost when dementia sets in. This is something that can be encouraged in joint groups too. For example, in one group in Bangor a retired art teacher was encouraged to put on his gown and resume his old role, giving the group an art class. Everyone did self-portraits, and the project team noticed that this man became more confident and articulate once in this role. He walked around saying positive things about everyone's work, and looked like a different man.

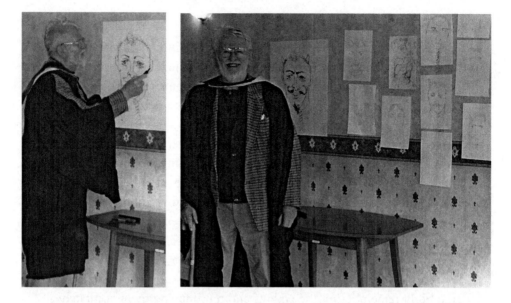

Figure 7.36a and b: A retired art teacher steps back into his familiar role to work with the group and experiences again his former confidence

Forming relationships

Project teams have noticed that participants with dementia seem to get closer to other people in the group in the Reminiscence Alone groups. When family carers are in the group, sometimes it seems that they don't feel the need to engage with others so much. People with dementia have also formed close links with workers and volunteers in the Reminiscence Alone groups.

A surprise phone call

The Bangor project leader reported that one of the people with dementia had found her name and home telephone number on a slip of paper near the phone when he was alone at home. He had evidently been reminded of the project and what fun he had joining in all the activities. This person was normally rather quiet, so the call was apparently out of character, but he spoke on the phone quite fluently for several minutes and was full of gratitude for the project. He said how much it had mattered to be part of the group and how it had improved the way he saw himself now and in the future.

Pacing activities

Facilitators have commented that activities may last for less time in Reminiscence Alone groups, perhaps because family members have a lot to contribute about their own memories in joint groups, whereas the contributions of people with dementia may be briefer.

SESSION 11: CELEBRATION (FOR REMINISCENCE ALONE GROUPS)

Objectives

- To draw together what has been explored throughout the project about each participant's life and character.

- To remember and celebrate the participants' stories.

- To remember and celebrate the work of the group.

The project team will need to do some preparation for this session. One way to organise it is for two members of the team to prepare a presentation about each participant with dementia.

Outline plan

Opening

As people arrive, greet them warmly and show the photos taken in the previous session (recording the 'still photographs' each group made based on memories of holidays and travel).

Main activities

1. Members of the project team present a short profile of each person with dementia, based on what has emerged in the previous sessions, selecting memorable material that can be celebrated and enjoyed. Invite group members not involved in the presentation to say what they liked about that person or comment on the stories they have shared or activities they have done together. It would be good to have a song connected with each person from one of the topics explored during the project.

Tea break: Remind people of what they said was their favourite childhood dish in the cooking session.

2. Use photos of the activities, to remind the participants of the different activities they have done together.

3. Make sure that everyone has some entries in their project books or wallets.

Work with individuals to decide what they would like to record about the project in the form of a drawing or short statement. It could be a general comment, a particular memory of one session, a tribute to a friend they have made on the project, or a card for the whole group with a message.

Closing

Make a large diagrammatic representation of the group, perhaps in the form of a tree or a round table or a bouquet of flowers and attach to it the offerings (see no. 3 above) of the people with dementia. Explore what everyone has said or drawn with the whole group and congratulate them on their contributions. Display the end result in a place where everyone can explore and enjoy it.

Give each member of the group a personal acknowledgement and farewell as the group closes.

REUNION SESSIONS

The RYCT project has run in many places in the UK and in Europe and in most cases participants do not want to stop meeting after the final session. They value the reminiscence activities, the opportunity to have fun together, the on-going contact with the other families and the new friendships they have made. Reunion groups, usually on a monthly basis where participants can come together and continue their reminiscence work, are an important follow-up to the project and have proved to be a highly desirable way of maintaining positive outcomes. This needs to be planned, a space allocated and staffing provided. Groups have often welcomed the chance to take more responsibility for organising and leading these reunion groups, but there will always be a need for professional coordination on matters of transport, communication and possibly organisation. Skilled reminiscence workers' continued input ensures the focus of the sessions and serves to coordinate the group's efforts.

In reunion sessions you can revisit previous themes, or explore other topics not covered in the original 12 sessions. Participants and the project team can work together to generate ideas, and you can devise activities to explore these themes based on your experience with the original sessions.

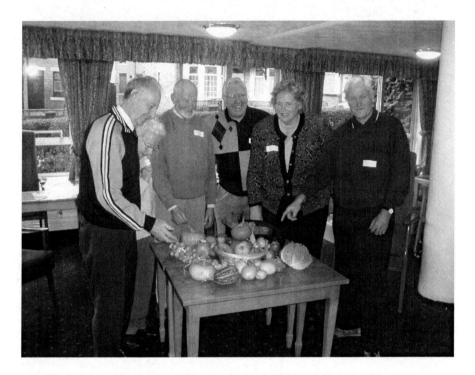

Figure 7.37: The Bradford group prepare a harvest festival display and celebration

Additional themes for reunion sessions

- Seasonal festivals

- Autumn memories

- Journeys to remember

- Fog and bad weather

- Trips to the cinema

- Grandparents

- Out in the country

- Hop-picking (or local equivalent)

- Anniversaries
- Grandchildren
- Favourite decades
- Being 21
- Where I was 50 years ago (or 30 or 20 or 10)
- Wartime experiences
- Evacuation
- Desert Island Discs
- Sports
- Health and illness / home remedies
- Retirement
- Housework
- Practical gardening, flowers and plants

Final Comments and Future Hopes

One of our tasks in writing this book has been to gather together accounts of Remembering Yesterday, Caring Today, and this has been a heartening experience. We have been reminded just how many families all over Europe have been touched by the project. We have re-read testimonies from carers and people with dementia, many emphasising how important it has been for them, particularly in providing the opportunity to have fun together, and an enjoyable social experience, at what is undoubtedly a very difficult time in their lives.

We have also looked through a great many photographs illustrating the high levels of engagement and animation so often generated in RYCT groups. Looking back over our experience of RYCT, we were reminded how often people who arrived looking tired and stressed left with their spirits lifted. We remembered the friendships made, some of which have lasted for years, and realised that making new friends at this stage in life can be very valuable for people with dementia, because new friends accept and enjoy them as they are now, without sadness or regret that they are no longer as they once were.

We hope that this book will be useful, both for people planning RYCT projects and for those who wish to bring a 'Remembering Yesterday' approach to the many different kinds of reminiscence work that can be done with people who have dementia. Inasmuch as the book is useful, thanks are due to all the people who have been involved in RYCT over the years. They have shared their ideas and experiences generously and given permission for their stories to be told.

Our hope for the RYCT *project* is that the new research will provide the evidence that is needed to convince service providers that it is a worthwhile intervention. Our hope for the RYCT *approach* is that it will continue to develop and inspire reminiscence work with people who have dementia, whether planned or spontaneous, with or without family members, individually or in groups, at home or elsewhere. It is a tried and tested approach, which we know has the potential to stimulate communication and conversation with people who are all too easily socially excluded and marginalised.

We would like to thank all those who have brought us to where we are now, and those who will take this work forward in future.

Perhaps we should leave the last word to a carer, Betty, aged 84, who was looking after a lifelong friend who had developed dementia. This is what she said:

> Taking part in this project has helped me to keep the true spirit of my friend alive, bringing back with a sense of pride the memory of the person she has been. And whilst I am now caring for my friend, it has been important to remember that once it was the other way round. The project has helped me to cope with our present difficulties by seeing them in the perspective of our long and very full lives.

Appendix: Useful Documents

CONTENTS

Handouts

Forms

Sample documents

GUIDELINES FOR RYCT PROJECT LEADERS AND VOLUNTEERS

We have identified in the following pages the essential ways of working that characterise the RYCT approach. To achieve these essentials, it is important that all members of the project team adopt the RYCT ethos, and make sure that it is reflected in how they respond to participants. When running a project it is not only *what* you do, but *how* you do it that is important to the success of the group. Project leaders can play an important part in helping volunteers see what is needed by modelling appropriate behaviour.

Supporting participants

- Greet participants individually and pay close attention to individual needs throughout the meetings. Make sure there are personal good-byes as well.

- Ensure that participants with dementia contribute fully and are given the time they need to speak for themselves. Allow extra time for people who are slow to express themselves and make good use of non-verbal communication.

- Value the contributions people make. Even if a story is clearly inaccurate or untrue (for example, someone claims a well-known poem as his or her own) be careful not to 'show people up' or embarrass them by drawing attention to mistakes, or showing that you don't believe that what they say is true.

- Be prepared to manage (as tactfully as you can) situations where particular individuals dominate the conversation, or carers speak for their relative with dementia unnecessarily, or try to correct their telling of a story.

- Notice if people are anxious or upset and support them discreetly within the group, or take them out of the room if this seems better.

Supporting family carers

- Be non-judgemental. Remember that seeing someone close to you change due to dementia is extremely distressing, and looking after that person on a daily basis can be very gruelling. People have different ways of coping.

- If carers have an urgent need to talk about caregiving problems and begin to discuss them in front of their person with dementia, take them somewhere private to do this. Give them some on the spot reassurance, but if possible arrange another time to talk at length if they need this, and then return to the group.

- Make sure that family carers experience the pleasure of reminiscence. Some may enjoy the opportunity to work in a group with other carers, while volunteers work with their relative with dementia.

- Praise carers for what they are doing in caring for their person with dementia.
- Remind carers that they are making an important contribution to the project.
- Be prepared so you are able to give carers information about dementia, and where they can go for support.

Good reminiscence practice

- Approach the activities with enthusiasm; join in with everything but make sure that your own contributions are not too lengthy – your main role must be to encourage and facilitate participants' contributions.
- Show that you have a genuine interest in people's stories by listening actively. Show in your body language that you are focusing on the speaker. Reflect back the stories as they emerge, and where appropriate, amplify contributions so that they can be shared by the whole group.
- Value humour, enjoyment, creativity.
- Respect people's right to tell their own story in their own way.
- Respect serious or painful memories, allowing people to express their feelings, whether positive or negative.
- Use the family members' knowledge of their relative with dementia and ideas from the project team to help find something that will involve everyone in some way in each session.

Building an inclusive group

- Use your 'people skills' to build a sense of belonging to the group.
- Express your delight in what people have contributed to the whole group.
- Point out common ground and connections between participants.
- Offer everyone opportunities to present something to the whole group, while making it clear that it is not compulsory.
- Give equal consideration to the needs of everyone in the group – and note that this does not mean treating everyone in the same way.
- If participants are critical or judgemental about certain group members, do not join in, even if you agree with their feelings.
- Behave in a non-judgemental and accepting manner towards participants, including staff and volunteers, and be understanding about people's failings and difficulties.
- Use every opportunity that arises to create a relaxed, convivial, enjoyable social occasion.

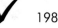

GROUP AGREEMENTS
The suggestions below can be discussed or changed by the group.

Confidentiality
- Are participants happy for things said in meetings to be discussed outside the group?

Respecting differences
- It is quite likely that participants will have very different views and opinions.
- Is it a good idea to take a non-judgemental attitude to one another's views?

Giving an equal share of time to each person
- Is everyone happy for facilitators to ask 'big talkers' to give others a chance to take their turn? If not, how will the group take responsibility for ensuring that this happens?
- How can we ensure that members of the group who need more time to assemble their thoughts are not rushed or sidelined by the rest of the group?

Expressing feelings
- Old memories can bring up strong feelings. Can we agree that it is quite all right for people to express their feelings?
- Can we agree to be supportive to anyone who is overcome by their emotions?

Photographs and video
- Photographs and videos are an important part of the group's history. Is everyone happy for photos to be taken and film to be shot?
- Are there any particular conditions you wish to attach to this?

ATTENDANCE RECORD

Participant	1	2	3	4	5	6	7	8	9	10	11	12	Total
Total													

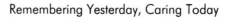

SESSION RECORD – PARTICIPANTS

Session no. . . . .   **Theme:** . . . .

Participant	P/C	Brief record of how they got on in the session / reason for absence

P = person with dementia
C = family carer

Records about participants

Briefly record your most significant observations of each participant, considering things such as how much interest and enjoyment they showed, how well they were able to communicate, any difficulties or setbacks, effects of mood, state of health, etc. For people who were absent, record reasons for absence.

SAMPLE COMPLETED SESSION RECORD

Session no. 1   Theme: Names and Origins

Participant	P/C	Brief record of how they got on in the session / reason for absence
Max K	P	Some apprehension, did settle OK
Faith K	C	Nervous but willing to give it a try
Richard F	P	Keen, lots of humour, aware of memory loss and talking of it
Jean F	C	Enjoyed herself, interacted well
Fred P	P	Some difficulty in settling to whole-group work
Pat P	C	Willing to participate but embarrassed by Fred's interruptions
James E	P	Enjoyed session and stayed very focused
Catherine E	C	Confident and supportive of activities
Nell R	P	Nervous, but very happy to reminisce at length
Simon T	C	Nervous, but settled into activity, slightly protective of Nell
Jim S	P	Interacted with volunteer well. Had not wanted to come, sense of gain observed at farewell time
Madeline S	C	Speaks for Jim. Watch possible jealousy over attention Jim gets?
Meg W	P	Hearing difficult. Singing engaged her. She will need one-to-one for reminiscence, very quiet voice – great ability in long-term memory
Pamela W	C	Supportive and enabling for her mother. Nervous.
James B	P	Sometimes engaged, but seems very sleepy, medication
Edna B	C	Very enthusiastic. Keen for James to have social contact

P = person with dementia
C = family carer

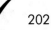

SESSION NOTES

Remembering Yesterday, Caring Today – Record of activities

Activities used today

Comments (what went well, what went not so well, who enjoyed what)

Points to consider in future sessions

SAMPLE COMPLETED SESSION NOTES

Session 6 – Weddings

Activities used today

We welcomed people as they came in and sat them on 'bride's or groom's side' of room laid out as church with two banks of seats. Tracy and Jim (Alice's husband) stood at front and got ready and the men and women copied them, hair, jackets, ring, makeup, dress, etc. Then we got the 'congregation' humming 'Sheep may safely graze' while waiting for the couple. We played out the wedding with Don and Eileen as couple and Fred as vicar, Jim as best man. 'Bit parts' for everyone else and all answered in role very appropriately. Couple had wishes from everyone and walked up aisle and back while we sang wedding march. Then we posed for wedding photos with whole group in picture.

Broke into small groups for discussion of wedding related objects at tables and wedding photos they'd brought in. Tea and special greetings and cake for Milly's 80th birthday (+cake/candles). After tea we had feedback from the groups on wedding stories. Hilarious tales, Edith telling her own. Dates of weddings written up on large paper and we made a list of the wedding presents people remembered.

Comments

- Atmosphere of fun and enjoyment.
- Everyone willing to join in activities and enter into role and situation.
- Star turns for everyone, Don and Mary as couple, May as Mum, Stephan as Dad, Sid and James as groom's mates, Alice as old flame, other aunties, etc. all in high good humour.
- Complicated coping with tea with no urn, but this managed well by extra Spanish students and volunteers.
- Stories were really interesting and people with dementia told their own.
- There are still problems between Milly and Sue (Mum and daughter, who drive each other mad).
- Comments by all the volunteers and workers that the group had gelled really well and seemed relaxed with one another.
- Edith's daughter missing, but lives 60 miles away and comes specially. Jean and David away for 2nd week running (Peter had heavy cold this week) but will come next time. The Campbells are still not coming. Don't know what to do about them.

Points for future sessions

The whole group enactment of the wedding worked really well giving everyone a chance to do something, high level of engagement, much humour and spontaneity. Definitely worth seeing how we can develop the pet show idea in next session.

HOPES AND FEARS (to be completed by participants, carers and volunteers)

This is your first meeting in a new group and you are probably wondering how things are going to turn out. We'd like you to record some of your thoughts and feelings.

What are your hopes?

What are your fears?

HOPES AND FEARS REVISITED

Please read the hopes and fears that you wrote down at the first meeting. Then think about what has happened since, and give us your comments.

Were your hopes realised?

Did any of the things you feared come about? If so, please explain.

REMEMBERING YESTERDAY, CARING TODAY – FINAL EVALUATION (to be completed by participants, carers and volunteers)

1. The session I most enjoyed and why

2. Something I remembered during one of the sessions which I have not thought about for ages

3. A surprise I had during the project

4. Something I learned

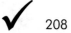

5. A new resolution, or a change I want to make

6. A friendship I made during the project

7. I would / would not recommend this project to a friend. Give reasons for your answer.

FOLLOWING THE RYCT APPROACH – CHECKLIST

(Ideally this should be filled in by an observer on a weekly session and the results relayed to the group leaders)

Communication

	Item	Y/N	Comments
1.	Was appropriate encouragement given to people with dementia to participate?		
2.	Was extra time allowed to enable people with dementia to gather their thoughts and speak?		
3.	Were team members indicating by their body language etc. that they were really listening?		
4.	Were team members responding appropriately to non-verbal communication, indicating how participants were feeling?		
5.	Were facilitators/team members showing they understood what people were saying by reflecting it back to them?		
6.	Did facilitators amplify and share individual contributions with whole group?		

7.	Did facilitators point out to the whole group connections between different participants' experience?		
8.	Was there space for both positive and negative feelings to be expressed?		
9.	Were ways found to involve everyone in the session?		
10.	Was the knowledge of family carers used to help to involve the people with dementia?		
11.	Were situations where family members dominated the conversation managed in a tactful manner?		
12.	Were situations where carers talked negatively about their relative in front of them well handled?		
13.	Did relatives have the opportunity to talk about problems in private?		
14.	Did family members work with other participants, and not exclusively with their own relative?		
15.	Were participants greeted individually?		
16.	Were name labels used in the session?		

Session structure and management

	Feature	Y/N	Comments
1.	Was there an opening (where participants are warmly welcomed, oriented to what is happening)?		
2.	Was there a warm-up activity including movement and optional physical contact?		
3.	Did the session have a chosen theme?		
4.	Was the session plan adapted in response to what was happening?		
5.	Was there a range of carefully chosen multi-sensory triggers appropriate to the theme (objects, images, music both live and recorded)?		
6.	Were one or more creative methods (other than just talking) used to explore memories, e.g. movement, song, improvisation, drawing?		
7.	Was the team working well to ensure that carers and people with dementia were all getting the support they needed throughout the session?		
8.	Was there a mixture of small-group and large-group work?		

9.	Was there feedback from the small groups to the main group?		
10.	Was the pacing of the different activities within the session appropriate?		
11.	Was there a closing where the work of the session was summed up and appreciated?		
12.	Did the closing involve participants thinking about the next session, including items they can bring in from home to help?		
13.	Were participants reminded to make use of the special books which the family members will keep?		
14.	Were good-byes personal and appreciative?		
15.	Were personal farewells given to everyone?		
16.	Was time allowed for the project team to reflect together, evaluating each session, noting individual responses?		
17.	Were these managed over all the sessions, if not in individual ones?		

CHECKLIST OF THEMES COVERED

	Theme	Y/N	Comments
1.	Introductions		
2.	Childhood and family life		
3.	Schooldays		
4.	Starting work and working lives		
5.	Going out and having fun		
6.	Weddings		
7.	Homes, gardens and animals		
8.	The next generation – babies and children		
9.	Food and cooking		
10.	Holidays and travel		
11.	Celebration		
12.	Rounding up and evaluation		

CONSENT FORM FOR PARTICIPATING FAMILIES TO USE PHOTOS AND VIDEO

There were photos and video taken during the group meetings. I give my consent for photos and video in which I appear to be used:

	Yes	No
to illustrate reports and articles about the project	☐	☐
in teaching and training sessions	☐	☐
in material used for teaching or training	☐	☐
in publicity (e.g. posters, newspapers, radio, TV)	☐	☐
in films, articles or books about reminiscence work	☐	☐
or caring for older people	☐	☐
in conference presentations	☐	☐
in exhibitions	☐	☐
on websites/Internet	☐	☐

I agree that photos and videos in which I appear can be used for the above purposes.

Participant. . . . .

Signature. . . . .

Date . . . .

SAMPLE WELCOMING LETTER

(to participants before sessions begin)

Dear

Welcome to the Remembering Yesterday, Caring Today Project. We look forward to working with you over the next few months.

Together we shall be exploring and sharing memories, getting to know about one another's lives, past and present, and having an enjoyable time.

There are 12 sessions at [e.g. 2–4 pm on Tuesdays]. They are based on key stages in life which most people will have experienced and which will, we hope, include everyone in the group. We have found that this chronological approach can also help families to take a longer view of their lives and undertake an informal 'life review'.

We may need to modify the outline timetable enclosed, but the list of dates and themes will give you some idea of what we shall talk about. It will also give you a chance to see what items you have at home (or stored with other family members) which you could bring along to the sessions.

At the first meeting we will give you a record book / document wallet in which to keep a record of the project if you wish. You can include photos, drawings, memories and comments from other people involved.

[Mention transport arrangements here and who to contact if unable to attend.]

We are really looking forward to working with you.

Relax and have fun!

SAMPLE INTRODUCTION TO THE PROJECT TEAM

An introduction to the people working on the project

ANNE SIMPSON is an experienced community arts and reminiscence worker. She has worked with many groups in the local area. Her particular interest is music and she loves playing songs from the 1930s. She lives in Widdicombe and has collected the life stories of many local farm workers and has made them into a book. She is looking forward to meeting the families involved in this project.

MARY JAMES works as an Occupational Therapist in the Community Mental Health Team for older people. She has used Reminiscence Therapy in the past and is always amazed at its ability to animate most people, no matter what their health needs are.

BILL SIMONS grew up in the area and has worked here all his life, starting off in Pike's Biscuits and ending up as a taxi driver. He really enjoyed the last project as he loves meeting people and sharing stories about the past.

KAREN WINSTON is a social work student. Her parents came to England from Jamaica, but she grew up in Cardiff. She wants to work with older people when she qualifies, and she is very interested in hearing stories about their lives.

SHEILA POLOWSKI has lived here since she married her husband Jim. She's worked in shops and offices. She remembers selling Pike's Biscuits when she worked evenings in the local corner shop! When her children grew up she worked for the council – first in planning, then social services. She retired last year.

References

Aldridge, D. (2000) *Music Therapy in Dementia Care*. London: Jessica Kingsley Publishers.

Allan, K. and Killick, J. (2000) 'Undiminished possibility: The arts in dementia care.' *Journal of Dementia Care 8*, 3, 16–17.

Alm, N., Dye, R., Gowans, G., Campbell, J., Astell, A. and Ellis, M. (2007) 'A communication support system for older people with dementia.' *Computer 40*, 5, 35–41.

Baldwin, C., Hope, T., Hughes, J., Jacoby, R. and Ziebland, S. (2005) *Making Difficult Decisions: The Experience of Caring for Someone with Dementia*. London: Alzheimer's Society.

Batson, P. (1998) 'Drama as therapy: Bringing memories to life.' *Journal of Dementia Care 6*, 4, 19–21.

Bell, V. and Troxel, D. (1997) *The Best Friends Approach to Alzheimer's Care*. Baltimore, MD: Health Professions Press.

Bell, V. and Troxel, D. (2001) *The Best Friends Staff: Building a Culture of Care in Alzheimer's Programs*. Baltimore, MD: Health Professions Press.

Bender, M., Bauckham, P. and Norris, A. (1999) *The Therapeutic Purposes of Reminiscence*. London: Sage.

Brooker, D. (2004) 'What is person-centred care?' *Reviews in Clinical Gerontology 13*, 3, 215–222.

Brooker, D. (2007) *Person-centred Dementia Care: Making Services Better*. London: Jessica Kingsley Publishers.

Brooker, D. and Duce, L. (2000) 'Well-being and activity in dementia: A comparison of group reminiscence, therapy, structured goal-directed group activity and unstructured time.' *Aging and Mental Health 4*, 4, 354–358.

Brooker, D, and Surr, C. (2005) *Dementia Care Mapping: Principles and Practice*. Bradford: University of Bradford.

Brooker, D. and Wolley, R. (2007) 'Enhancing opportunities for people living with dementia: The development of a blueprint for a sustainable activity-based model of care.' *Aging and Mental Health 11*, 4, 371–383.

Bruce, E. (1998) 'Reminiscence and family carers.' In P. Schweitzer (ed.) *Reminiscence in Dementia Care*. London: Age Exchange.

Bruce, E. and Schweitzer, P. (2008) 'Working with life history.' In B. Bowers and D. Downs (eds) *Excellence in Dementia Care: Principles and Practice*. Maidenhead: Open University Press.

Bruce, E., Hodgson, S. and Schweitzer, P. (1999) *Reminiscing with People with Dementia: A Handbook for Carers*. London: Age Exchange (for the European Reminiscence Network).

Butler, R.N. (1963) 'The life review: an interpretation of reminiscence in the aged.' *Psychiatry 26*, 65–76.

Chaudhury, H. (2003) 'Remembering home through art.' *Alzheimer's Care Quarterly 4*, 2, 119–124.

Cheston, R. and Bender, M. (2000) *Understanding Dementia: The Man with the Worried Eyes*. London: Jessica Kingsley Publishers.

Coaten, R. (2001) 'Exploring reminiscence through dance and movement.' *Journal of Dementia Care 9*, 5, 19–22.

Cohen-Mansfield, J. (2005) 'Nonpharmacological interventions for people with dementia.' *Alzheimer's Care Quarterly 6*, 2, 129–145.

DSDC Wales (2002) *Services for People with Dementia in Wales. Report No. 1: Residential and Nursing Home Care in Wales.* Bangor: Dementia Services Development Centre.

Gibson, F. (1998) *Reminiscence and Recall: A Practical Guide to Reminiscence Work*, second edition. London: Age Concern.

Gibson, F. (2004) *The Past in the Present: Using Reminiscence in Health and Social Care.* Baltimore, MD: Health Professions Press.

Goldsmith, M. (1996) *Hearing the Voice of People with Dementia: Opportunities and Obstacles.* London: Jessica Kingsley Publishers.

Greenyer, J. (2003) 'Music and memories.' *Journal of Dementia Care 11*, 1, 8.

Haight, B.K. and Haight, B.S. (2007) *The Handbook of Structured Life Review.* Baltimore: Health Professions Press.

Hallbierg, I.R., Holst, G., Nordmark, A. and Edberg, A. (1995) 'Co-operation during morning care between nurses and severely demented institutionalised patients.' *Clinical Nursing Research 4*, 1, 78–104.

Heathcote, J. (2007) *Memories are Made of This: Reminiscence Activities for Person-centred Care.* London: Alzheimer's Society.

Johns, C. (2000) *Becoming a reflective practitioner.* Oxford: Blackwell Science.

Killick, J. and Allan, K. (1999a) 'The arts in dementia care: Tapping a rich resource.' *Journal of Dementia Care 7*, 4, 35–38.

Killick, J. and Allan, K. (1999b) 'The arts in dementia care: Touching the human spirit.' *Journal of Dementia Care 7*, 5, 33–37.

Killick, J. and Allan, K. (2001) *Communication and the Care of People with Dementia.* Buckingham: Open University Press.

Kitwood, T. (1997) *Dementia Reconsidered.* Buckingham: Open University Press.

Knocker, S. (2002) *The Alzheimer's Society Book of Activities.* London: Alzheimer's Society.

Moos, I. and Bjorn, A. (2006) 'Use of the life story in the institutional care of people with dementia: A review of intervention studies.' *Ageing and Society 26*, 3, 431–454.

Naess, L. (1998) 'Reminiscence work with people with dementia.' In P. Schweitzer (ed.) *Reminiscence in Dementia Care.* London: Age Exchange.

NICE (2007) *A NICE-SCIE Guideline on Supporting People with Dementia and their Carers in Health and Social Care, CG42.* London: British Psychological Society and Gaskell.

Nolan, M., Grant, G. and Keady, J. (1996) *Understanding Family Care.* Buckingham: Open University Press.

Peak, J.S. and Cheston, R. (2002) 'Using simulated presence therapy with people with dementia.' *Aging and Mental Health 6*, 1, 77–81.

Perrin, T. and May, H. (2000) *Wellbeing in Dementia: An Approach for Therapists and Carers.* Edinburgh: Churchill Livingstone.

Powell, J. (2000) *Care to Communicate: Helping the Older Person with Dementia.* London: Hawker Publications.

Robb, M., Barrett, S., Komaromy, C. and Rogers, A. (2004) *Communication, Relationships and Care: A Reader.* New York: Routledge.

Sabat, S.R. (2001) *The Experience of Alzheimer's Disease: Life through a Tangled Veil.* Oxford: Blackwell.

Schweitzer, P. (1998) *Reminiscence in Dementia Care.* London: Age Exchange (for the European Reminiscence Network).

Schweitzer, P. (2004) *Mapping Memories: Reminiscence with Ethnic Minority Elders.* London: Age Exchange.

Schweitzer, P. (2007) 'Use of drama in outreach work and in dementia care.' In P. Schweitzer *Reminiscence Theatre: Making Theatre from Memories*. London: Jessica Kingsley Publishers.

Sheard, D. (2004) 'Bringing relationships into the heart of dementia care.' *Journal of Dementia Care 12*, 4, 22–24.

Violets-Gibson, M. (2004) 'Dance and movement therapy for people with severe dementia.' In S. Evans and J. Garner (eds) *Talking Over the Years*. London: Routledge.

Ward, R., Vass, A.A., Aggarwall, N., Garfield, C. and Cyloyk, C. (2005) 'What is dementia care? 1. Dementia is communication.' *Journal of Dementia Care 13*, 6, 16–19.

Woodhead, H. (2004) 'Mind the generation gap.' *Journal of Dementia Care 12*, 2, 12.

Woods, B. (2003) 'Evidence-based practice in psychosocial intervention in early dementia: How can it be achieved?' *Aging and Mental Health 7*, 1, 5–6.

Woods, B., Spector, A., Jones, C., Orrell, M. and Davis, S. (2005) *Reminiscence Therapy for Dementia* (Cochrane Review). London: Cochrane Database of Systematic Reviews.

Woods, R.T. (2002) 'Non-pharmacological techniques.' In N. Qizilbash, L. Schneider, H. Chui *et al.* (eds) *Evidence-based Dementia Practice*. Oxford: Blackwell Science.

Woods, R.T. and McKiernan, F. (1995) 'Evaluating the impact of reminiscence in older people with dementia.' In B.T. Haight and J. Webster (eds) *The Art and Science of Reminiscence: Theory, Research, Methods and Applications*. Washington, DC: Taylor and Francis.

Wuest, J., Erikson, P.K. and Stern, P.N. (1994) 'Becoming strangers: The changing family caregiving relationship in Alzheimer's disease.' *Journal of Advanced Nursing 20*, 3, 437–443.

Yale, R. (1999) 'Support groups and other services for individuals with early stage Alzheimer's disease.' *Generations 23*, 3, 57–61.

PRACTICAL GUIDES

Dementia care

Bell, V. and Troxel, D. (1997) *The Best Friends Approach to Alzheimer's Care*. Baltimore, MD: Health Professions Press.

Brooker, D. (2007) *Person-centred Dementia Care: Making Services Better*. London: Jessica Kingsley Publishers.

Kitwood, T. and Bredin, K. (1992) *Person to Person: A Guide to the Care of Those with Failing Mental Powers*. Loughton: Gale.

Knocker, S. (2002) *The Alzheimer's Society Book of Activities*. London: Alzheimer's Society.

Reminiscence

Bruce, E., Hodgson, S. and Schweitzer, P. (1999) *Reminiscing with People with Dementia: A Handbook for Carers*. London: Age Exchange.

Gibson, F. (2006) *Reminiscence and Recall: A Practical Guide to Reminiscence Work*. London: Age Concern.

Heathcote, J. (2007) *Memories are Made of This: Reminiscence Activities for Person-centred Care*. London: Alzheimer's Society.

Osborn, C. (1993) *The Reminiscence Handbook*. London: Age Exchange.

Schweitzer, P. (1998) *Reminiscence in Dementia Care*. London: Age Exchange (for the European Reminiscence Network).

Schweitzer, P. (2004) *Mapping Memories: Reminiscence with Ethnic Minority Elders*. London: Age Exchange.

Subject Index

Author Index